GETTING PREGNANT SIMPLY
AND
RESOLVING
RECURRENT MISCARRIAGE

A CLINICIAN'S ADVICE BASED ON 50-YEARS EXPERIENCE AND MANY SUCCESSES OF WORKING WITH INFERTILE COUPLES

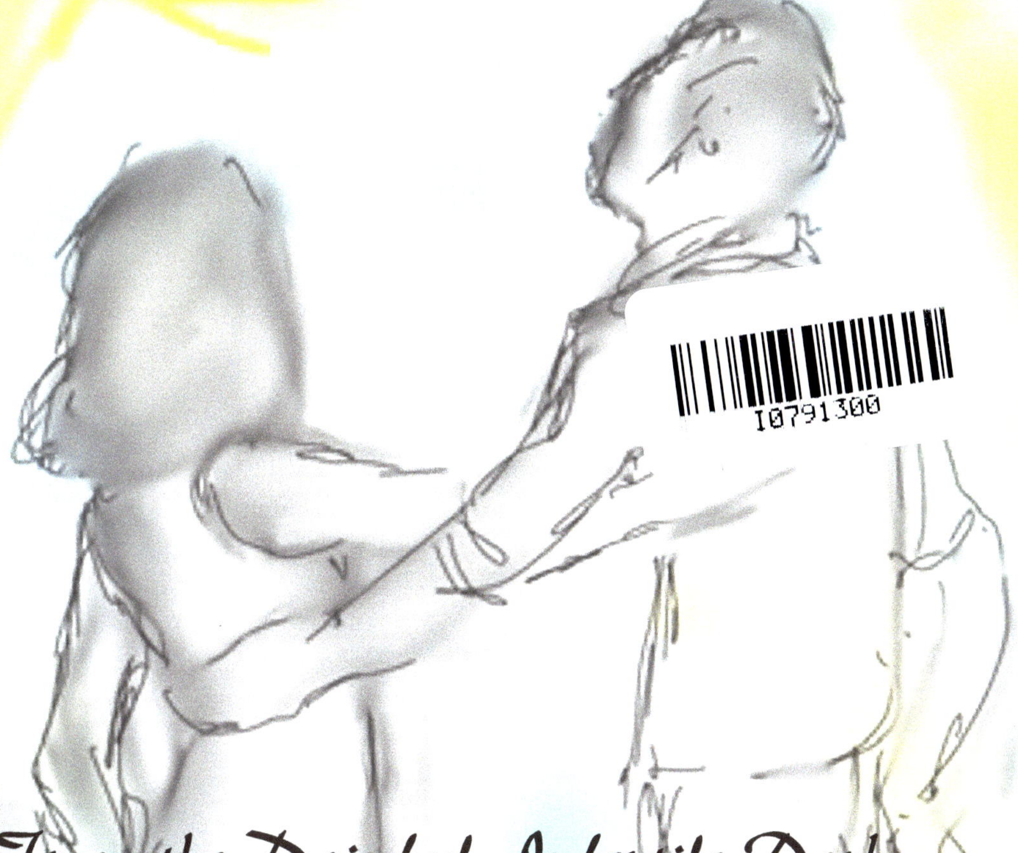

From the Painful, Infertile Dark-

Seeking the Light…

Dr. Brian M. Cohen, Mb., ChB., M.D. (Post-Doctoral)

PAGE PUBLISHING, INC.
Conneaut Lake, PA

First originally published by Page Publishing 2021

The opinions expressed in this booklet are purely those of the author. They do not formally direct specific treatment options or methods. These thoughts should be reviewed by all couples with their physicians, who will direct their own treatment strategies. This booklet explains basic methods and should be a guide to provide reassuring direction in your care. These diagnosis and treatment techniques were formulated by synthesis of evidence based writing in the literature over the past fifty years. They were applied to my own patients, under my care.

ISBN 978-1-6624-4352-7 (pbk)
ISBN 978-1-6624-4353-4 (digital)

This book transparently describes the principles of diagnosis and treatment of patients with infertility and solutions to be explored in those with recurrent miscarriage in an environment charged with assisted reproductive technology. This volume provides the fundamental knowledge to assist in the possibility of having a more simple therapy that may help them have a viable pregnancy without the need for assisted reproductive technologies.

To contact the author, please email him at <u>bmcohenmd@gmail.com</u>.

The artwork was painted by Mary Jane Alexander, a well-known British painter from Camberley, Surrey. Born in Zimbabwe, she immigrated to England in 1977. She has worked with many dance companies, and a series of her paintings based on Fosse was shown at the Prince of Wales Theatre—West End. She has had multiple residencies and commissioned work throughout the United Kingdom. Her work is presently on show in many significant British Galleries. Find her work at <u>https://www.maryjanealexander.co.uk</u>.

Dear Dr. Cohen,

I wanted to send you a note to make sure you know what you've meant to me and to our family. I always tell people that Cece, now three, is here on this earth because of G-d and Dr. Cohen. You were such a source of hope for me after losing three babies in a row. You always believed that I was capable of carrying another baby and were the only one who helped to really figure out why I was miscarrying in the first place. You took a personal interest in my situation and gave me your full attention and heart. You offered personalized care, specific to my situation and to my body—and I know that is why I did not miscarry Cece.

Elizabeth and Shahnia were amazing as well, so positive and encouraging. Cece is truly such a complete source of joy, and I know that G-d meant for her to be here, and he meant for you to be my doctor.

Thank you with love,
AM

With twenty years of experience counseling couples struggling with infertility, I have been disappointed time and again to hear how quickly they are unwittingly placed on the fast track to **ART** and specifically **IVF**. Unfortunately, the fertility process has been commercialized and this often causes innocent couples to invest hundreds of thousands of dollars, in addition to time, energy, and pain unnecessarily. Contrary to the "protocols" that many of the popular clinics adhere to, fertility treatment is ***not*** a "one-size-fits-all" and couples must be seen and heard to be successful.

Dr. Brian Cohen understands this and utilized his outstanding medical expertise, tenacious attention to detail, passionate love for every person, and a deep understanding of the human spirit to help bring children to thousands of couples that had all but given up hope. Dr. Cohen's holistic approach combined with cutting-edge technology and the belief that he is "just a messenger of G-d" brought us our three miracles and changed our lives forever.

After fifty years in the trenches, Dr. Cohen shares the simple facts needed to understand infertility in this concise booklet.

This is a must-have for any couple that dreams of building a family.

—Rebbitzn SRB

Foreword

I met Dr. Brian Cohen almost thirty-five years ago. I was a green, freshly minted obstetrician gynecologist just beginning to realize that there was far more to learn about the complexities of reproductive function than I had been taught during my training.

Dr. Cohen taught me to question everything, listen to my patients, and always, always keep their well-being central to any treatment plan. We have worked together in the many years since that time to promote best practices in reproductive health and care. Over the years, there have been many spectacular advances in reproductive science—including in vitro fertilization (IVF), intracytoplasmic sperm injection (ICSI) just to name a few—but the fundamental principles are unchanged. Dr. Cohen had a dedicated team and offered all these technologies within the scope of his infertility practice. The principle, however, was that all care must be individualized, directed toward the patient's goals and designed to do the right thing for the right patient at the right time.

This book is an attempt to give couples the resources and information they need to be able to find the right care, and to participate with their clinician in figuring out the right decisions at the right time. Dr. Cohen's dedication to "what's right" to listening, learning, and constantly adjusting therapy to provide the best possible outcomes for couples has been clear throughout his career and has resulted in this booklet.

On a personal note, I have Dr. Cohen to thank for my two fantastic grandsons. His brilliant approach to the management of couples with recurrent miscarriage is unique. He has fought "the system" for years to bring specialized care to couples with this problem. This booklet provides the basics for couples facing difficulties achieving pregnancy (infertility) as well as for those who have no trouble conceiving but are unable to continue a pregnancy to term (recurrent losses).

Read this with the confidence and trust that the information is accurate, up-to-date, and written for people facing tough situations in their reproductive lives. Listen to the pearls of wisdom within this booklet and use the information to guide you through your journey.

With many thanks to Dr. Cohen and his team for my wonderful grandchildren—and for the opportunity to participate in this work.

—Barbara Levy, MD, FACOG, FACS, FRCOG (hon)
La Jolla, CA

Acknowledgments

My beloved wife of fifty-five years, Rose, who made my life and love of practicing medicine a steady romance. To all my family members whose multiple sacrifices made it possible for me to always be there for my patients.

To my teachers, colleagues, nurses, and students whose teamwork and teaching continued to maintain a caring and excellent clinical practice. To all my NFC and Cohen Center staff: coworkers, MDs, Scientists, RNs, and organizational and secretarial staff. Each of you made a significant contribution of knowledge, team spirit, clinical application, and compassionate caring. To my patients whose questions always ensured that I did my daily reading to keep up with the latest facts. To my daughter and Head Nurse Shahnia Cohen. Her clinical brilliance and compassionate caring for our patients was a major force with me for twenty-six years. To my executive director and business manager Elizabeth Dominguez who was at my side for twenty-eight years and made my practice of medicine pure joy. Barbara Levy, MD—whose constructive criticism and editorial assistance helped elevate the content of this booklet. David E. Martin, MD, who together with his staff and aesthetically beautiful office, afforded our patients a warm, compassionate, and uplifting experience for the last fifteen years of my practice.

To Dr. Benjamin Leader, MD, PhD, who provided much insight in the interpretation of NK cell testing. Keri Stern who, given a pack of sheets, brilliantly created this lovely manuscript.

I hold you all in esteem. I salute and gratefully thank you all.

—Brian M. Cohen, MB, ChB, MD (Post Doctoral)

Getting Pregnant Simply

A CLINICIAN'S ADVICE BASED ON 50 YEARS EXPERIENCE AND MANY SUCCESSES OF WORKING WITH INFERTILE COUPLES

By: Dr. Brian M. Cohen, Mb., ChB., M.D.

(Post-Doctoral)

Table of Contents

GETTING PREGNANT SIMPLY

CHAPTER ONE	Introduction	15
CHAPTER TWO	Basic Anatomy, Sexuality, and Fundamentals of Human Reproduction	18
CHAPTER THREE	Physiology of the Menstrual Cycle	24
CHAPTER FOUR	"The Fertile Period" of a Menstrual Cycle	28
CHAPTER FIVE	Conscientiously Answering The Physician Questionnaire	30
CHAPTER SIX	The Female	31
CHAPTER SEVEN	The Male	36
CHAPTER EIGHT	Fundamentals of Treatment	38
CHAPTER NINE	Additional Testing in the Complicated Patient	41
CHAPTER TEN	Unexplained Infertility	43
CHAPTER ELEVEN	Summary and Conclusions	46

Chapter One

INTRODUCTION

This booklet is written in the interest of and to support modern young couples who seek treatment for the problem of infertility.

It advises patients of simple, diagnostic, and treatment methods for primary infertility. The primary objective is that all couples facing the problem of infertility should have a basic understanding of how each partner is checked, simple options of treatment, and the fundamental information to empower them to receive the most optimal treatment available. When fully investigated, and simple treatment measures fail, they are encouraged to seek assisted reproductive technology. Hopefully, this booklet will enlighten couples with understanding of the fundamental issues that should be applied, to optimize their chances of success in their pursuit of pregnancy.

We have treated all patients with the utmost respect for their personal faith, be it Muslim, Hindi, Buddhist, Baha'i, Christian, or Jewish.

At the present time, both Orthodox Jewish and Catholic couples are encouraged to seek fundamental treatment that, if at all possible, does not immediately progress to assisted reproductive technology (***ART***) and in vitro fertilization (***IVF***).

The booklet defines the fundamentals of diagnosis and treatment in both male and female. It proposes a formula to accomplish pregnancy in the simplest yet detailed, most straightforward, personalized, individual, and efficacious effective manner.

If a couple has completed the fundamental treatment outlined in the following sections and it has not been successful, then ***ART*** and ***IVF*** are advised for those whose religion allows them to proceed.

In other couples, a few more attempts at conception may be made to attempt pregnancy and may yet be successful without resorting to assisted reproductive technology, but the success rate becomes progressively lower.

Overall, the sentiment of this book is designed to equip and empower couples who seek fertility treatment, with the fundamental knowledge of reproductive care, so that they can play an active role in their management.

Once adequately informed, couples understand the various problems that are affecting their fertility. They can ask their specific questions and seek a physician who will treat their individual problems, respectful of their religious boundaries.

The current state of infertility treatment in many centers around the US tends to advocate pushing couples into the early pursuit of in vitro fertilization in many centers. There has to be a legitimate basic treatment before proceeding to assisted reproductive technology, particularly in young and modest living, monogamous couples. It makes more medical as well as financial sense to exhaust controlled and limited basic treatment options before proceeding to *ART*.

When seeking conception, a couple should be aware of the fundamentals of human reproduction. These are important basics to understand as couples work toward pregnancy. Imparting such knowledge to them equips and empowers the couple to have some understating and to be aware of the questions to ask the physician.

Most young men and women with no previous major issues such as prior infections, multiple partners or known disorders, such as diabetes, should conceive within approximately three cycles after completing the recommended tests, and aggressive pursuit of appropriate noninvasive hormonal treatment.

If ***three optimized cycles have been unsuccessful,*** the couple and their physician would be equipped with the knowledge to clearly understand their individual problems. They may then proceed to *ART* tailored to their specific needs. Couples should never lose hope as even after completing all treatments, approximately 16 percent will still conceive. This is well documented as treatment-independent pregnancy.

DEFINITION OF INFERTILITY:

Couples aged 35 years or older, who have not conceived over six months with unprotected intercourse. Younger couples less than 35 years old, who have not conceived over twelve month of unprotected intercourse.

These are the basic rules but there are clearly exceptions. There are some couples who have significant, known, underlying medical issues. For them earlier intervention or advancing to assisted reproductive technology is warranted.

In general terms, the cause of infertility is related to the female in 40% of cases, the male in 40% of the cases, and 20% related to issues involving both partners. Thus, it is essential that we review the basic issues of sex and reproductive function of both partners.

Furthermore, to maximize conception and the chances of achieving pregnancy, it is essential that each woman is aware of her individual fertile time, during the menstrual cycle. This varies considerably and is dependent on the length of woman's specific cycle. There are several period-tracking apps available for iOS and Android that can also be very helpful (FLO, Clue, Ovia, Natural Cycles to name just a few).

$Chapter Two$

BASIC ANATOMY, SEXUALITY, AND FUNDAMENTALS OF HUMAN REPRODUCTION

THE MALE—SEXUALITY

After puberty and maturation, the pituitary gland (the small "master gland" that sits just underneath the lower portion of the brain) releases two main sex hormones, **FSH** and **LH**. These hormones stimulate the testicles to produce sperm and to make testosterone. The main male sex hormone, testosterone, stimulates the male sex drive and sperm production.

Libido (another word for sex drive) is driven by testosterone but also influenced by cultural and environmental factors. These may be visual, olfactory, auditory, or tactile. Certain parts of the body called erogenous zones are more sensitive than others.

Excitatory events result in increased desire and associated erection, with penile enlargement and engorgement. When an appropriate partner is available, this will result in initiation of sexual activity. The male seeking stimulation (foreplay) and ultimately penetration of the female vagina-intercourse.

Once excited and proceeding to intercourse, the male will then continue pelvic movements until involuntary loss of control and orgasm occur and with a sense of pleasure as sperm is ejaculated into the vagina. The amount of semen fluid emitted (which is made up of the sperm and surrounding liquid) will be dependent on the length of abstinence (how long since the most recent ejaculation) and the amount of excitement in an individual sexual encounter.

MALE ANATOMY AND BASE FUNCTIONS

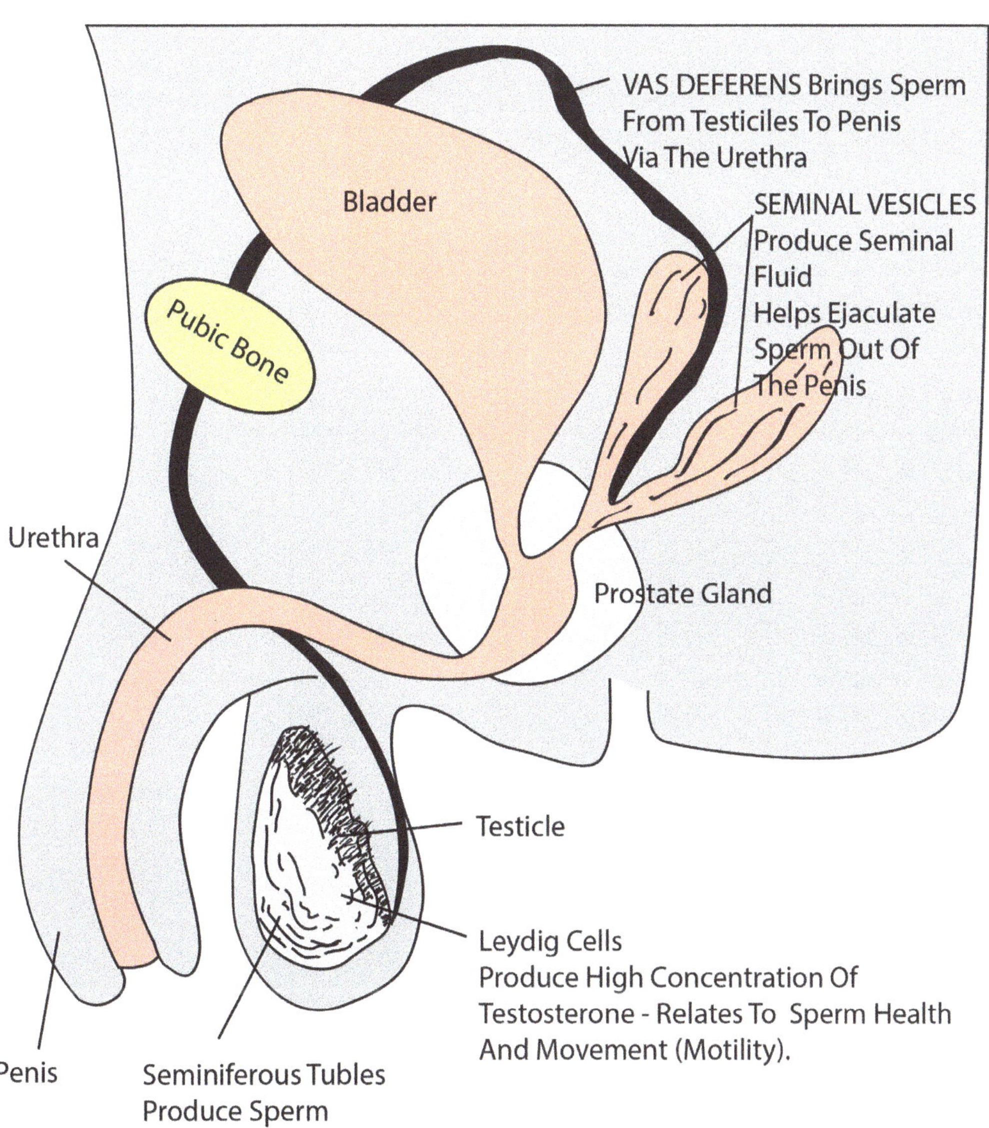

BASIC HORMONES OF MALE REPRODUCTIVE SYSTEM

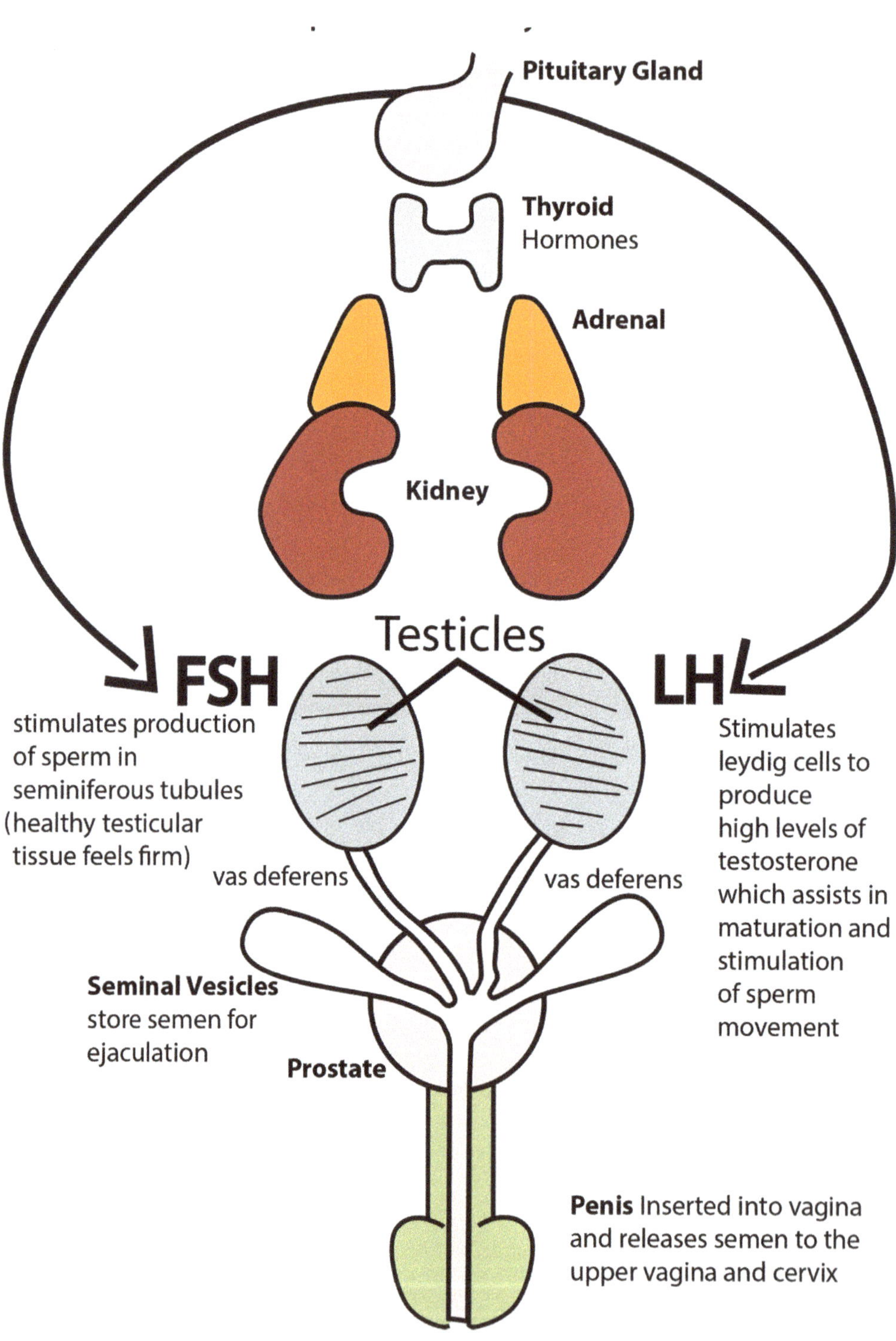

THE FEMALE—SEXUALITY

The hormones of the human female have a far more intricate and rhythmic pattern. These are organized with the goal of orchestrating the stimulation of adequate ovulation (release of an egg from the ovary) at midcycle, fourteen days before the next menstruation. For women with longer cycles, the fertile time won't be in the "middle" of the cycle but rather 14 days before the next expected period. Female libido (sex drive) can be of various forms but clearly is far more subtle and influenced by many external factors including fatigue, emotional connection, and anxiety among others. Unlike the male, the female is not always concerned with thoughts of sex, but is more sensitive and responsive to the overall situation including the male's concerns, kindness, and advances in pursuing her interest.

The female is also influenced by cultural, religious, endogenous situations, relationship, and environmental factors.

The female may also have somewhat cyclical needs, finding that she is more responsive at different times in the menstrual cycle.

As in the male, the female is excited by all of her senses and also has erogenous zones with varying intensities in different places of her body including her inner thighs, breasts, pubic area, and, in particular, the vaginal opening nipples and clitoris.

When excited, the breasts are somewhat swollen and sensitive and the pelvic organs are engorged, also with increased sensitivity. If adequately stimulated in foreplay, the female will then be in a phase of pleasurable excitation that she may experience, and may be orgasmic as a culmination. The female may have orgasms repeatedly with little time in between; whereas, the male will usually have a refractory phase when he cannot be stimulated, but will become responsive again once this refractory phase has passed. The refractory phase may last for minutes to hours in the young and hours to days in the older male.

TRANSVERSE SECTION OF FEMALE REPRODUCTIVE ORGANS

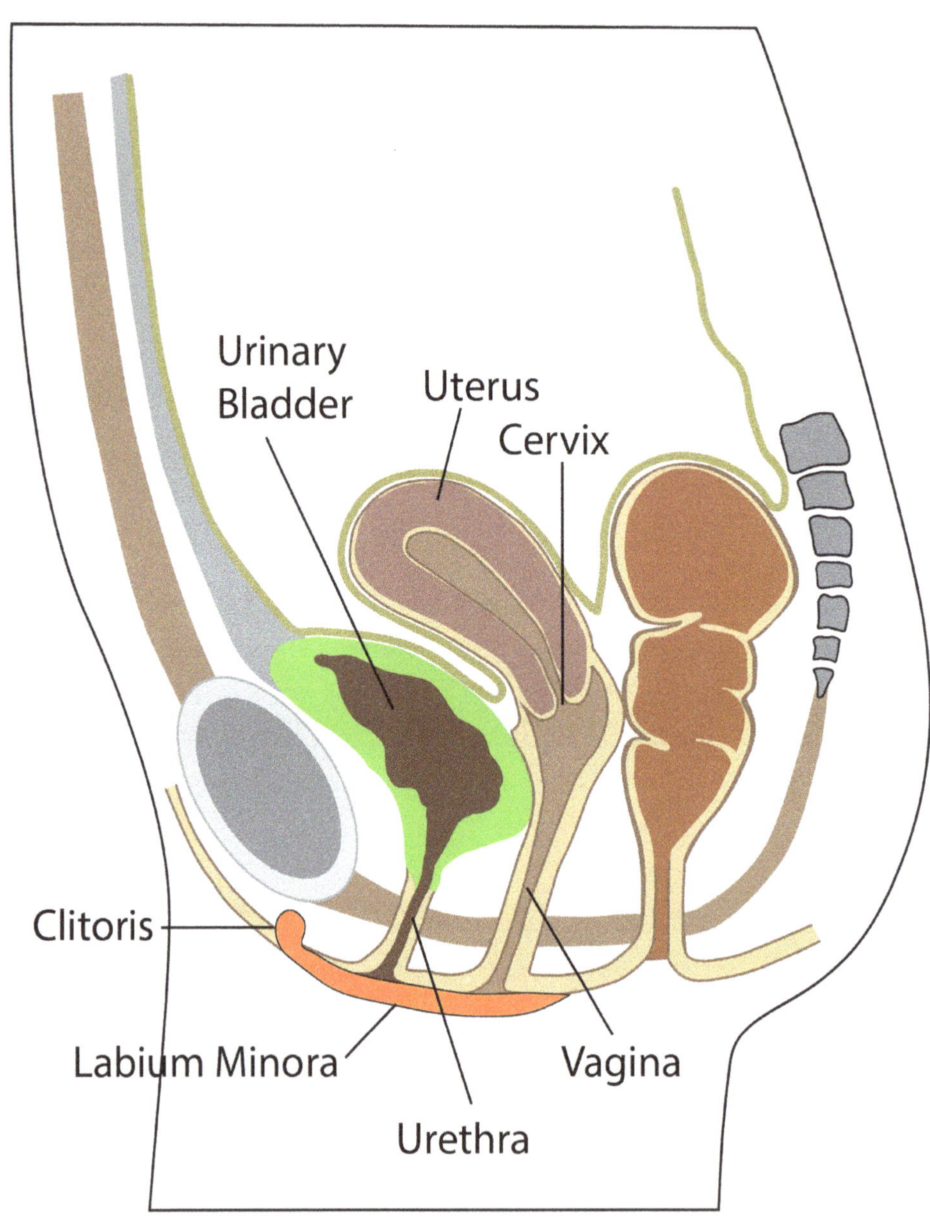

FRONTAL VIEW OF VAGINA AND PERINEUM

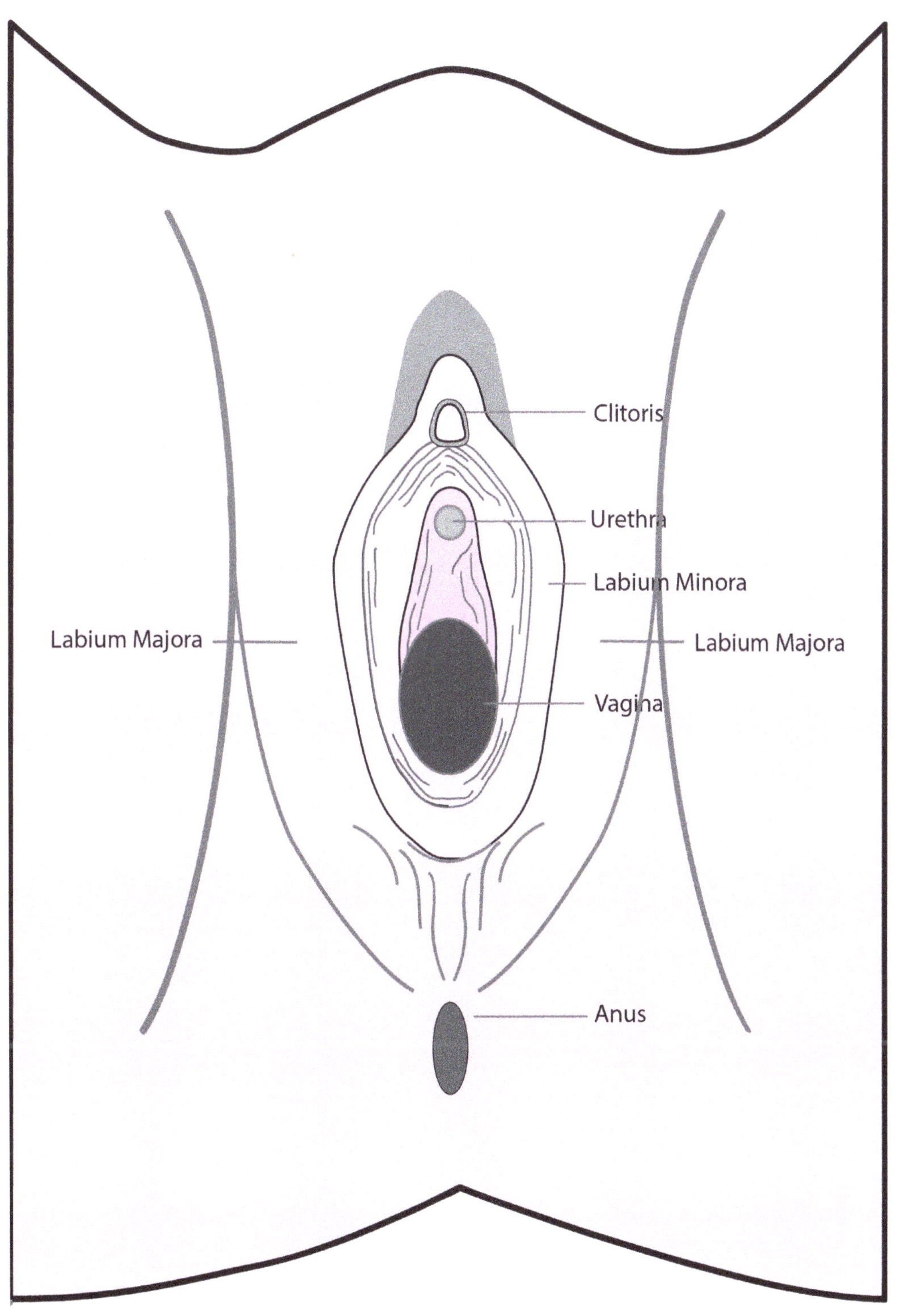

Chapter Three

PHYSIOLOGY OF THE MENSTRUAL CYCLE

Menstruation symbolizes the loss of the inner lining of the uterus that had been prepared to receive a fertilized egg for conception at midcycle. With the onset of menstruation, a new cycle begins with the secretion of **FSH** and small amounts of **LH** from the pituitary gland. These hormones stimulate the ovaries to produce follicles, one of which will mature to be the primordial or dominant follicle, at ovulation. This follicle will burst (ovulation) to release a mature egg for fertilization.

HORMONES OF MENSTRUAL CYCLE

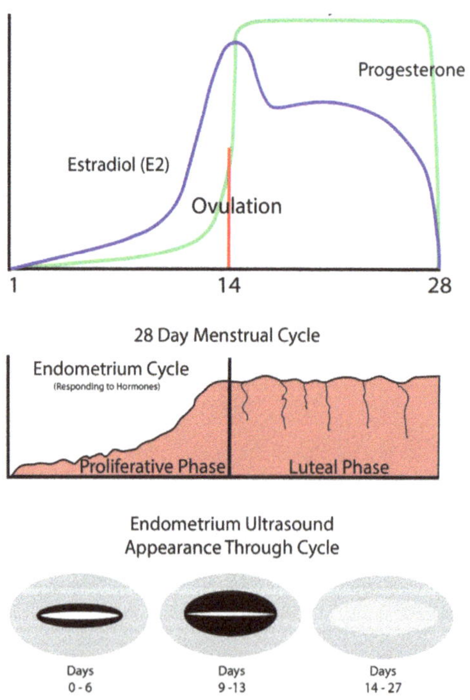

HORMONAL CONTROL OF FEMALE MENSTRUAL CYCLE

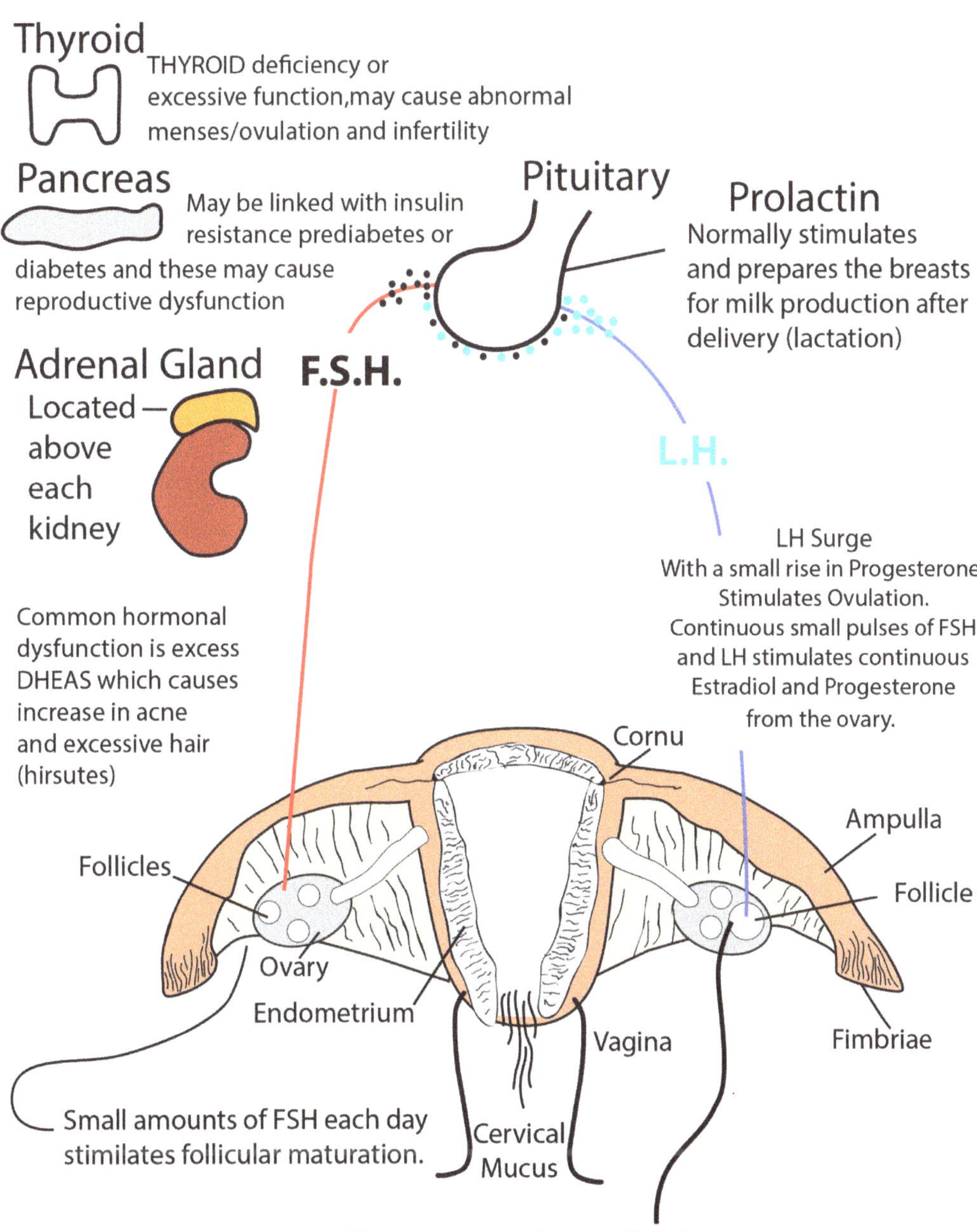

The estrogen (estradiol) content of the blood results from the development of the dominant follicle and escalation of estrogen production immediately prior to ovulation. At this time, following a minimal rise of progesterone, the pituitary gland releases a surge of *LH*, which among other functions, assists ovulation by stimulating enzymes, which soften the capsule of the ovary, to help the lead follicle rupture and release the egg in a ball of cells called the cumulus. The egg within these cells sticks on the surface of the ovary.

The *LH* surge also stimulates hormonal production of progesterone and estrogen from the corpus luteum (the residual cyst left after release of the egg) from the ovary.

Approaching midcycle, and a few days before peaking at ovulation, the cervix secretes abundant thin mucus which is highly stretchable. Under the electron microscope, the mucus is now in open columns and stimulates the sperm to enter through the cervix, swim through the uterine cavity, and accumulate in the ampulla of the fallopian tubes to await the arrival of the egg.

Sex at midcycle results in many healthy activated sperm, being present in the fallopian tube within 45 to 60 seconds from the time they entered the vagina and cervical mucus. Simultaneously, the fallopian tubes are stimulated by the rising estrogen. The tubes become engorged, and their muscles are activated to pull the end of the tubes to the surface of the ovary. The fine, delicate ends of the tube (fimbriae) work to collect the egg and transmit it into the outer third of the fallopian tube.

The sperm usually fertilize the egg in the outer part of the tube. Once fertilization has taken place, the fertilized egg divides into and has become eight cells by the third day. By the fifth day, it has divided into a ball of cells (morula). The cells continue to divide into a blastocyst which is then transported by contraction of the tube into the waiting uterus.

In the uterus, the blastocyst continues development for two to three days when implantation should occur into the uterine lining (endometrium). Once implantation has occurred, the trophoblast (specialized cells of the embryo) produces *HCG* (the pregnancy hormone), and the uterine lining is now referred to as decidua. It is at this point that a sensitive pregnancy test will turn positive.

THE SECOND HALF OF THE FEMALE CYCLE IS CONSISTENTLY 14 DAYS.

If fertilization and implantation have occurred, and the woman has conceived, she will not have her period. The pregnancy hormone (*HCG*) will continue to stimulate the ovary to make progesterone and estrogen from the corpus luteum. This organ, formed in the follicle that ruptured in the ovary, is normally programmed to function for only 14 days, unless pregnancy occurs. The *HCG* of pregnancy then continues to stimulate and maintain the corpus luteum. If the patient does not conceive and pregnancy has not occurred, the corpus luteum ceases to function and the hormones progesterone and estradiol drop, resulting in menstruation. Bleeding generally means there was no conception, and indicates the loss of the lining of the uterus.

Chapter Four

"THE FERTILE PERIOD" OF A MENSTRUAL CYCLE

From what was written above it is clear that, in a **28-day cycle**, the fertile time will be approximately day 12 until day 16. If the patient's cycle is longer, e.g,. **31 days,** it would be 14 days before the 31st day, that is, days 15 to 19, and if the patient's cycle is **35 days**, her fertile time would be day 19 to 23. This information is extremely important so that a couple is aware of their individual fertile time in the menstrual cycle.

Alternative methods of timing sexual activity at the peak of fertile time in the menstrual cycle can be gauged digitally estimated by checking the quality of cervical mucus, monitoring first morning "basal" temperature or on by using an **LH** (ovulation) surge guide testing kit that looks for the hormone **LH** in urine, obtained daily from a woman's urine.

THE FERTILE TIME OF A MENSTUAL CYCLE.

Always +/- 12–14 Days From The Next Menses 28 Day Cycle

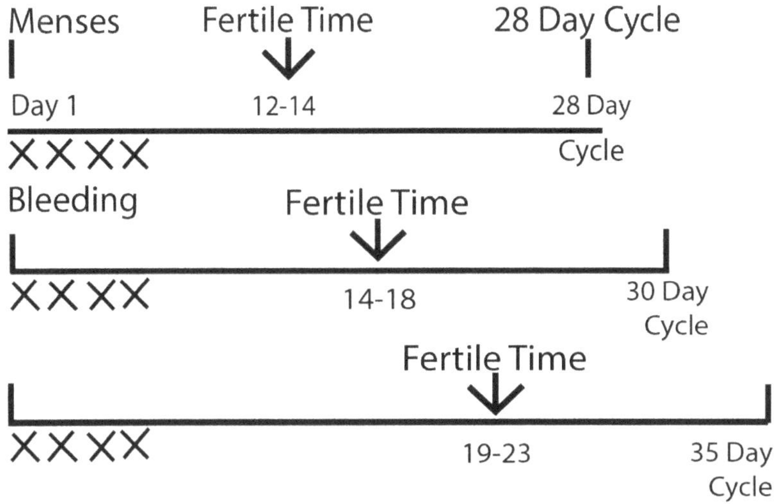

The old-fashioned way of looking at a temperature graph can give the couples a guideline regarding sexual timing. Then, having watched the early morning temperature (taken on awakening) throughout a menstrual cycle, helps the couples know when the temperature will rise after ovulation occurs. In future cycles, the couple would be able to predict the best time for sex and conception.

In Jewish couples, halachically, the period of Nida (abstinence), ends seven days after the end of menstrual bleeding. This is consistent with an average of 12 to 13 days from the first day of a 28 day menstrual cycle. Thus when a couple resume sexual activity after Nida, they commence sexual activity at the peak fertile time of the cycle.

Unrelated to Nida, it is important for each couple to be aware of their maximal time of fertility (as indicated above), knowing the length of an individual woman's menstrual cycle, and her peak fertile time.

Chapter Five

CONSCIENTIOUSLY ANSWERING THE PHYSICIAN QUESTIONNAIRE

If you are sent a questionnaire before your first visit, it is important to answer all questions. These answers provide pointers (clues) to the physician and assist in focusing your appointment on specific matters that may affect either partner. Using this information, your doctor can target certain issues in either partner and concentrate the history and physical examination, seeking a correlation with the personal points you have highlighted in the questionnaire.

See Glossary for Questionnaires.

Pending your responses, the questionnaire should in principal help to illuminate the specific factors that should be pursued in either partner.

When a couple first visits a fertility specialist (***Reproductive Endocrinologist***), they should expect the following sequence of events: a detailed history, physical examination, and blood testing.

Chapter Six

THE FEMALE

HISTORY

Your physician needs to be aware if there is a personal or family history of:

> *Diabetes*
> *Thyroid disease*
> *Adrenal dysfunction*
> *Excess male hormone*
> *PCOS (polycystic ovarian syndrome)*
> *Auto-immune disorders including:*
> Lupus
> Asthma
> Psoriasis
> Eczema
> Ulcerative colitis (IBS)
> Crohn's Disease
> Endometriosis
> *Chromosomal disorders*
> *Recurrent miscarriage*

Excessive smoking of tobacco, marijuana, or much alcohol, and participating in minimal exercise or excessive exercise are all factors that may all be contributors to infertility.

Your ***BMI*** reflects your body fat, and if your ***BMI*** is extremely low or high, this is important. Body fat is an active organ of the body and stores the building blocks for many important reproductive hormones.

MENSTRUAL PAIN

Understanding the severity, timing, and site of pain with your periods provides vital information—raising suspicion of endometriosis.

The amount of bleeding at/or during your period is also extremely important. Average blood loss would require 8 to 12 pads, or 12 to 18 tampons, with mild to moderate staining. Please inform your doctor if you have ***very short periods or extremely heavy periods***; these symptoms may signal problems in the uterus.

Advise your physician if you have acne, excess hair, irregular periods, minimal bleeding, or no periods, and if you have no pain or severe pain or no breast tenderness or severe tenderness before your period, or if you have milk from your breasts, as these are all important factors to be shared.

Your doctor should be made aware of any history of prior abdominal or pelvic surgery, or previous dilatation and curettage (D & C). Other important concerns that need to be discussed are your sexuality, including your libido, general sexual function including any pain on intercourse, aversion to sex, failure of lubrication, and/or prior abuse or molestation.

Though it may be uncomfortable, it is extremely important to tell your doctor about any issues within your relationship—either emotional or sexual.

EXAMINATION

Pelvic examination allows assessment of your pelvic organs (vagina, cervix, and the size and location of your uterus).

Pelvic ultrasound (usually with a small probe placed in the vagina) defines the size, shape, and the inner lining of the uterus (endometrium). Serial ultrasounds across the menstrual cycle allow observation of the changes in the lining of the uterus as you progress through your typical cycle.

LABORATORY TESTS

Blood Hormones:
  Pituitary—FSH, LH, Prolactin
  Thyroid (TSH, T3, T4, FTI)
  Adrenal—DHEAS
  Ovarian—AMH (Anti-Mullerian Hormone)
  Estradiol, progesterone, and when indicated, testosterone and free testosterone

Primordial Follicle Count (PFC)
  Follicles in the ovary observed on ultrasound early in the menstrual cycle. A low *PFC* usually corresponds to a low *AMH*, and vice versa.

Blood Chemistry
  Glucose/Insulin ratio HBA^{1C} (If indicated)
  Electrolytes—sodium, potassium, chloride
  Urea, creatinine
  Liver functions—Bilirubin, Alkaline phosphatase, *SGPT*, *SGOT*

Muscle Enzyme
  Creatinine phosphokinase (patients on statins)

Hematology
  Red blood cells
  White blood cells
  Hemoglobin,
  Hematocrit
  Platelets

Chromosomal and Genetic Analysis

The physician will select specific testing in relation to your period, family history and the findings at physical examination.

DIAGNOSTIC TESTS

Hysterosalpingogram (HSG)

An X-ray assessment of the uterine lining that is performed just after menstruation and prior to ovulation. The doctor will place a loaded syringe of fluid (with a rubber cork) against the cervix or slip a small tube up through the cervix to flush out the fallopian tubes with an oil contrast medium. *HSG* has been associated with higher pregnancy rates during the cycle of and subsequent two cycles after this procedure.

Hydrotubation (Tubal Irrigation)

Fluid is passed through the uterus and flushes out the fallopian tubes, as done at an *HSG*, but is completed in the physician's office with no X-rays.

Hysterosonogram

Passing fluid through the uterus and the fallopian tubes with ultrasound visualization of the fluid in the uterus and passing through the tubes.

Hysterosalpingogram (HSG), Hydrotubation, or hysterosonogram

(if not done within the past six months) is performed as a therapeutic event. This optimizes treatment during the first and subsequant two treatment cycles. ***Each of these procedures flush out the fallopian tubes.***

Endometrial Biopsy

In this procedure, a tiny suction tube is slipped into the uterus to obtain a piece (small sample) of the endometrial lining. This procedure may be timed on varying days of the menstrual cycle seeking different information.

Hysteroscopy

A tiny telescope is passed through the cervix to look into the uterine cavity. If performed in the operating room, uterine repair can be completed. The uterus and fallopian tube uterine openings are checked at hysteroscopy. It allows one to see the size, shape, surface, and any abnormalities, such *as severe paleness (less blood flow)*, polyps, adhesions, and evidence of chronic infection.

Laparoscopy

A surgical procedure looking into the abdomen and pelvis through the umbilicus (belly button). The surgeon can repair or treat any abnormalities noted in the abdomen. This procedure includes observation of the gall bladder, upper abdominal organs, and the appendix. A detailed examination of the uterus, ovaries, benign or malignant masses, and the fallopian tubes, and whether or not they are open or closed.

The surgeon checks for congenital abnormalities, inflammatory changes, adhesions, and endometriosis.

Demonstrating *tubal patency* (open tubes) is accomplished using dilute blue dye—indigo carmine, which is passed through the uterus and exits the ends of the tubes into the pelvis.

The diagnosis of *endometriosis* is most commonly made at laparoscopy, which remains the gold standard for assessing the presence or absence of this disorder. Patients with moderate to severe endometriosis constitute a significant number of those who will be positive for Natural Killer cells. This is not surprising, for the illness is known to have an immunological basis amongst other causes.

Other than timed endometrial biopsy, all fertility-promoting procedures are performed in the first half of the menstrual cycle, *days 8–10.*

NOTE: Those considered to have "long tubes" at Hysterosalpingogram or Laparoscopy should rest for approximately 40 minutes twice a day on their abdomen during their fertile time after intercourse. (Irrespective of their sexual position at this time.) This helps the long tubes fall down to the surface of the ovary and may assist in egg pick up.

Chapter Seven

THE MALE

HISTORY

Inform your doctor if you participate in excessive smoking of tobacco and marijuana, alcohol intake, and use of hormones. This includes testosterone or anabolic steroids (as a pill, patch, or injection). If you visit the sauna or hot tub, or are exposed to toxic chemicals or insecticides at work, please advise your doctor.

The doctor should know if there is a family history of chromosomal disorders or congenital abnormalities, problems with your libido, testicular or penile pain, erectile dysfunction, or orgasmic disorders should be mentioned. All drug use including over the counter and prescription medications should be disclosed.

EXAMINATION

A general examination is completed first. Local testicular examination confirms firmness of the healthy testicular tissue. Very soft testicles are a sign of prior testicular damage.

In the standing male, there should be no varicocele (large veins) between the lower abdomen and the scrotum containing the testicles.

LABORATORY TESTS

To accommodate Orthodox Jews and Catholics, ***indirect assessment*** of the presence and quality of semen is accomplished by timed, midcycle, postcoital testing. The cervical mucus is abundant, thin, and stretchable at this time. The woman is asked to come to the doctor's office soon after sexual intercourse without showering or bathing. Some mucus is withdrawn from the cervical canal, and placed on a warmed slide and cover slip.

Cold slides or cover slips can cause ***cold shock*** to the sperm. This decreases the motility, and may even cause them not to move at all.

The numbers of sperm are counted (per high-powered field) on the slide. Their speed of forward progression (***SFP***) shows how quickly they move across the slide. This is scored from 0 to 4, for example 1, 1+, 2, 2+, 3, etc. If this test does not appear to be adequate, e.g., less than 5 sperm per field, and hardly moving, then one must proceed to a ***formal semen analysis***. The semen specimen is usually obtained by masturbation or partner manipulation and delivered to the laboratory within an hour of collection.

In religious patients, a special condom is issued with a perforation in it. The semen is obtained at intercourse and transferred from the condom into a sterile specimen container by the patient. This should be delivered to the laboratory within an hour.

For a semen analysis, a certified technician assesses the volume, numbers (millions per ml), the total in millions, and the motility and speed of forward progression.

The sperm's morphology (size and shape) is checked by viewing the head, neck, and tail in 200 sperms. The percentage of perfectly normal looking sperm is known as the ***Kruger*** score. The number of immature sperm, presence or absence of white cells, and the presence or absence of fructose, which should be found in normal semen, are all identified. To have a normal Kruger score, 4–5% of the sperm should be perfectly normal.

Chapter Eight

FUNDAMENTALS OF TREATMENT

To secure pregnancy, the concept of establishing "fertile cycles" is essential. One must confirm adequate ovulation with adequate luteal phase function. This demands detailed observation, but activating perfect cycles is necessary to accomplish pregnancy.

THE CONCEPT OF ADEQUATE, FERTILIZABLE, HEALTHY OVULATION

What does this mean?

The concept of adequate quality (hormonally and physically) of fertilizable, healthy ovulation is a must.

Ovulation implies ***release of an egg from the surface of an ovary***, irrespective of the adequacy of hormone levels present.

Adequate levels of hormones are also required to prime the organs of reproduction; The cervical mucus to allow sperm optimal transit into the tubes; the uterus to receive a fertilized egg; the tubes to collect the egg and transport the embryo.

This includes making sure there is a healthy uterine lining, normal tubal function, and normal ovarian hormonal responses.

This adequate production of hormones from a healthy developing follicle—with ***adequate estrogen*** before ovulation facilitates optimal and timely tubal function. The corpus luteum should produce ***adequate estrogen and progesterone*** after ovulation (during the final fourteen days of the cycle) and maintain an adequate uterine lining and the best environment for implantation of the embryo.

Adequate estrogen and progesterone are also necessary for appropriate growth, function, and viable progress of the embryo during the first twelve weeks (trimester) of pregnancy.

Commitment to the biological concept of adequate ovulation fertilization and functional normality for conception and establishing a healthy pregnancy is a must.

The goal is that excluding a ***major genetic or chromosomal issue***, which is an age related handicap, one must ensure a healthy functional hormonal environment to maximize the chance of having a viable pregnancy.

A twenty-eight-year-old may have a risk of miscarriage of 15–20%, whereas in a forty-year-old, this risk rises to 40%. One cannot change these age-related chromosomal/genetic odds. However, in principle, if all the factors in the female and the male are normal, or corrected, the highest probability and chance of a healthy first twelve weeks of pregnancy are accomplished.

This is achieved by augmenting naturally an adequate "stimulation of ovulation" and following through with boosting of corpus luteum function during the luteal phase. If conception occurs, hormonal maintenance is also continued for the first twelve weeks of pregnancy.

In order to optimize the hormonal environment, the medical team will determine an ***individualized protocol*** for each patient.

This may include any of the following: a tailored dose of **HMG** (human menopausal gonadotropin) in every cycle; supplementation with estradiol before ovulation (if needed), midcycle use of HCG (human chorionic gonadotropin), washed intrauterine insemination, supplementation of the luteal phase of the cycle with the individualized required doses of progesterone and estradiol. This all facilitates a "perfect cycle," each month, in every patient.

When the patient is first seen, if they have not conceived during the past six months (for those over thirty-five) or twelve months (for those younger than thirty-five), they should proceed to this active but noninvasive treatment.

If the patient is forty or older, one aims at early **ART** and **IVF**, unless not permitted on religious grounds.

I prefer to call this ***augmented supraphysiological "fertile" ovulation***. Augmented ovulation is done to ensure adequate hormonal ovulation with or without washed intrauterine insemination (***WIUI***). Adequate hormonal support is also ensured during the second half (luteal phase) of the menstrual cycle.

Note: We continued to use the technique of washed intrauterine hydro insemination as first instituted forty years ago; 3–4 ml of culture medium containing the washed sperm are injected via the cleansed cervix into the fallopian tubes. Anecdotally, our impression was that this method optimized our pregnancy rate and was preferable to minimal volume, intrauterine catheter placement.

Chapter Nine

ADDITIONAL TESTING IN THE COMPLICATED PATIENT

In the female, one would correct hormonal abnormalities.

Elevation of **Prolactin** should be lowered with a dopamine agonist. **Abnormal Thyroid Function**, over or under active, is corrected with the appropriate medication.

An elevated **DHEAS** (from the adrenal gland) should be controlled during the first ten days of a menstrual cycle with dexamethasone 0.5 to 0.75 mg daily (pending body weight). Dexamethasone should be taken in the morning with a small piece of a sandwich—as it can cause stomach irritation, which may lead to ulceration and/or bleeding. Dexamethasone may cause significant loss of sodium, potassium, and calcium, so adding these supplements to the diet is a good way to avoid depletion.

The patient with a significantly elevated **ANA** (anti-nuclear antibody) is given prednisone 5 mg, twice a day, from day 2 of the cycle, and 5 mg, three times a day, after ovulation. If she becomes pregnant, this is continued through twenty weeks of pregnancy and is then tapered off by slow reduction of dosage at that time.

BLOOD CLOTTING ISSUES

Anti-phospholipid antibodies, protein S, Leiden factor, sticky platelet syndrome, and elevated anti-thyroid antibodies are treated with heparin and aspirin (81mg). There are many different protocols for commencing heparin and changing to enoxaparin in early pregnancy. We replaced heparin with enoxaparin at twelve weeks.

For ***Insulin Resistance***, the primary treatment is to optimize diet and exercise. If this fails, controlling the insulin may require an ultra-low carbohydrate diet or a medication such as glucophage, to normalize the high insulin/glucose ratio. It is also a positive way to assist the patient to lose weight, coincidentally lowering the insulin, provides a healthy environment which preserves egg quality in a woman with this problem.

When all these hormonal disorders have been controlled, one is ready to proceed to controlled ovarian hyperstimulation.

Chapter Ten

UNEXPLAINED INFERTILITY

Few couples were described as having "unexplained infertility" or no detectable cause for their problem.

In our practice, the unexplained comprised less than 5% of our patients, for we completed **comprehensive testing** and verified the causes in each partner.

Invariably, there were three to four cumulative reasons why a couple was not conceiving. There were factors documented in both husband and wife. When they would proceed to in vitro fertilization (**IVF**), their problems and abnormalities were clearly defined, as detailed diagnostic testing had been completed. They, therefore, proceeded to **IVF** with **known abnormal factors corrected** and an optimal chance of success.

NATURAL KILLER CELLS

Positive natural killer cells (**NKC**) require treatment, and modern laboratories will indicate whether **intralipid** or **gammaglobulin** will be successful as an intravenous therapy to lower and normalize **NK** cell levels present.

If abnormal high numbers of natural killer cells are present, these must be lowered **at least ten days before embryo transfer or conception**. The treatment is repeated on diagnosis of pregnancy.

As the pregnancy proceeds, the **NKC** cell test is repeated monthly, to assess if further infusions are necessary. The patient is treated every month if the test remains positive until thirty-three to thirty-four weeks of gestation.

Once there are two negative tests, further **NK** cell treatment is discontinued.

A third of the patients have a positive **NKC** test through twelve weeks of pregnancy, a third to eighteen to twenty-four weeks, and a third are repeatedly positive until term.

Although controversial, having had, over the past thirty-five years, well over one thousand viable babies in women with an average of five prior failures or losses, at an 82% success rate, I have no doubt that this **NKC** cell diagnosis and its treatment are an ***important scientific and clinical entity***. Sadly, significant numbers of patients presented to us after five to thirteen failures to conceive or miscarriage, many of these women were diagnosed with positive natural killer cells, when tested. With treatment, they joined the 80% plus success category with a viable infant. Other than 3.3% headaches and 2.2% short-term rapid heart rate during infusion, there were no significant reactions to the gammaglobulin.

All patients treated were IgA antibody negative. A critical safety factor. (See advanced reading regarding natural killer cells in glossary.)

FERTILITY MEDICATIONS

The American College of **OB/GYN** recommends the use of letrazole as the first line of treatment. This drug is given day 3 to 7 of the menstrual cycle. From five days later, the couple has intercourse and repeats sexual activity every other day. This medication accomplished an acceptable pregnancy rate with least multiple pregnancies.

The second drug, Clomiphene Citrate, has been the most commonly used in the past fifty years. It is successful in effecting ovulation, but it's relatively low incidence of pregnancy (9–15%), and a high chance of miscarriage (30%), risk of tubal pregnancy (5% to 10%), and multiple pregnancies (5–8%) were the main drawbacks to this medication.

My experience of the past 50 years has taught me that ***"the most natural stimulation" is accomplished using human menopausal gonadotropins (HMG).*** These are supplemented with estrogen and progesterone, where necessary, and combined with washed intrauterine insemination. This is followed by administration of estrogen and adequate progesterone, if needed, to ensure an adequate second half of the cycle. The key issue in using **HMG** is understanding the art of using the medication later in the cycle. The injections (**HMG**) even half an ampoule, are begun once there is a dominant follicle. This is usually day 6–8 of a twenty-eight-day cyscle and day 11–13 in patients with a thirty-one- to thirty-three-day cycle. This includes patients with polycystic ovaries (**PCOS**) and irregular cycles. Starting with half an ampoule, we accomplished single follicle ovulation in over 90% of these women and two to three follicles in 10%, 5% of whom had twins.

If the patient has not conceived during three of these HMG-stimulated cycles—the couples are prepared for in vitro fertilization, pending their faith and religious practice.

All patients who have "unexplained infertility," even after failed **IVF**, should not lose hope, for as many as 16% have been reported to conceive independent of active treatment. *Treatment independent pregnancy* is well-known and multiple reasons have been offered as to why it occurs.

Chapter Eleven

SUMMARY AND CONCLUSIONS

This booklet has been written to provide guidelines of simple, fundamental diagnosis, and treatment options for couples who have infertility.

These directions should guide the couple regarding the basics of testing and treatment methods. This information educates and empowers the couple with knowledge of these important concepts.

Once they have reviewed these concepts, the couple should be capable of asking their physician pertinent questions. If repeatedly rebuffed by the clinician, they should understand that it is time to find an alternative fertility physician.

The key issue is that the doctor should demonstrate his/her commitment and compassion to assess the two partners as an ***individual and unique*** couple. Time should be allotted to facilitate the diagnosis of your individual problem. You should be aware of the causes and options for your care. This knowledge enables you to make informed choices in treatment.

Hearing stories of multiple failed cycles, with unexplained infertility, multiple miscarriages, and minimal testing of blood clotting and immunological issues (including natural killer cells) suggests the need for ***more diagnostic testing*** in these patients.

The doctor should be able to ***identify the causes of your problem*** (often one or two issues in either partner), attend to them, and hopefully assist you in a positive outcome for your treatment.

May all your dreams and wishes come true, and may you be blessed to have the baby you so earnestly desire.

Resolving Recurrent Miscarriage

A CLINICIAN'S PERSONAL PERSPECTIVE

By: Dr. Brian M. Cohen, Mb., ChB., M.D.

(Post-Doctoral)

This dissertation reflects a "specialized practice" and reviews fifty years of clinical experience treating patients presenting with recurrent miscarriage. The data may be skewed by the fact that most patients had an average of five miscarriages and had seen two to three doctors before presenting.

Table of Contents

RESOLVING RECURRENT MISCARRIAGE

INTRODUCTION — 51

COMMON CAUSES — 51
    CHROMOSOMAL
    DNA FRAGMENTATION

OVULATORY DYSFUNCTION ASSOCIATIONS — 52
    ELEVATED PROLACTIN
    ELEVATED DHEAS
    ELEVATED TESTOSTERONE

LUTEAL PHASE DEFECT — 53

COMMONLY UNRECOGNIZED UTERINE ANOMALIES — 54

OPERATIVE PROTOCOLS FOR INTRAUTERINE SURGERY — 54

ASSESSING POSTSURGICAL UTERINE FUNCTION WITH A SIMULATED TREATMENT CYCLE — 55

DETAILS OF ASSESSMENT AND CORRECTION OF FUNDAL ISCHEMIA — 56

HEMATOLOGY AND BLOOD CLOTTING — 57

IMMUNOLOGY AND NATURAL KILLER CELLS — 59

IMPORTANCE OF THE DQ ALPHA PHENOTYPE — 60

INSTITUTING MONO-FOLLICULAR OVULATION   **62**

CERVICAL INCOMPETENCE   **63**

GLOSSARY   **67**

Introduction

The etiology of miscarriage is multiple, usually involving combinations of causes in the female and sometimes associated with causes originating in the male.

COMMON CLINICAL CAUSES OF RECURRENT MISCARRIAGE

Cervical infection—5%

It was not uncommon to find patients who had prior mycoplasma, ureaplasma, bacterial, or chlamydial infections.

This was one of the first tests completed to ensure that both partners did not need treatment for any of these infections. Unless allergic or a record of prior failure with this antibiotic, both partners were treated with doxycycline 100 mgs twice a day for ten days. Bacterial vaginosis, if diagnosed, was treated appropriately with clindamycin or metronidazole.

CHROMOSOMAL ABNORMALITIES

less than 3%positives were found in preconceptual testing,+_ 15% in the abortus of those less than thirty-five years of age and +_40% in women over thirty-eight years.

In the young patients, this appeared to be a random nonrecurring event. If it was recurrent (e.g., Robertsonian translocation or another persistent chromosomal anomaly), the incidence of same was only 2–3%.

Robertsonian translocation meant that the patient would lose three of four future pregnancies. To ensure viability of the residual 25%, it was critical to diagnose any additional factors and manage them appropriately. Nowadays this would be a classic indication for IVF with genetic diagnosis and embryo selection if religiously permissible.

In older patients over thirty-eight years of age, chromosomal abnormalities were picked up in approximately 40% of the aborted tissue.

This means that to have a viable outcome in the pregnancies of chromosomal normal embryos, the other causes of recurrent miscarriage that may also apply in the individual patient must be investigated and treated in a thorough and detailed fashion.

Male patients with severe Teratazoospermia (Kruger scores less than 4%), severe asthenospermia and olgospermia were sent for chromosomal analysis, but the pickup rate for aneuploidy in these patients was only 7%.

Testing for *DNA* fragmentation revealed a positive rate in only 2% of our male partners.

As we had observed a significant improvement in prior male patients, with DNA fragmentation using the supplements in *PROXEED* (L-carnitine fumarate 1,7G, L-arnitine-1G, and 0.5 Gacetyl-L-carnitine) was prescribed. Five hundred milligrams of vitamin C, 2,500 international units (IUs) of B12, 2,500 IUs of B complex, plus one milligram of folic acid were also given daily to all new male partners for three months from when they were first seen.

All *female* partners were given vitamin B_{12} (2500ius), vitamin D2000ius, vitamin B complex, folic acid 1.8 mgs, and vitamin C 500 mgs/as routine daily supplements.

FEMALE FACTORS

OVULATORY DYSFUNCTION

The hormonal factors that cause ovulatory dysfunction and/or luteal phase deficiency. These multiple defects include hypothalamic-pituitary, thyroid adrenal and ovarian dysfunction.

A most important factor in the history was marked *hypomenorrhea* with scanty bleeding over two to three days.

Minimal bleeding was suggested by the patient using a total, of three to five tampons or two to three pads for her whole menses. This was commonly found in patients' post hypothalamic-pituitary amenorrhea or oligo menorrhea, and those with prolonged exposure to birth control pills, progestin intrauterine devices, or subcutaneous progestin implants. Depot medroxyprogesterone was also included in this group.

Hyperprolactinemia was corrected with bromocryptine.

Hyperandrogenism was corrected when present.

Elevated DHEAS was suppressed during the first ten days of the menstrual cycle with Dexamethasone 0.5 to 0.75 mgs pending body weight.

Low or excessive thyroid function are treated appropriately.

Those presenting with **serum testosterone levels persistently above 100ng/ml** were first treated, with a minimum sixty-day course of an estrogen dominant birth control pill.

Significant drops in serum testosterone to normal levels were confirmed before proceeding to attempt conception. This ruled out a **testosterone-producing tumor**, and facilitated the normal expression of estrogen and progesterone in subsequent menstrual cycles.

Low levels of estrogen and progesterone associated with luteal phase deficiency were commonly seen in these patients before lowering testosterone, in the manner described. This enabled adequate elevation and function of estrogen and progesterone in the luteal phase of subsequent cycles for approximately three months.

LUTEAL PHASE DEFECT

This was diagnosed in many patients, based on a midluteal progesterone less than or equal to 8 ng/ml or the findings at late cycle (greater than 26 days) endometrial biopsy.

It was related to: older age, prior prolonged hormonal contraception, hypothalamic pituitary ovarian dysfunction, a high-stress lifestyle, prolonged nutritional disorders, participation in excessive exercise, and low **BMI** patients.

The negative effects of prolonged hormonal contraception on the endometrium were suspected when observing an **echogenic uterine fundus** on vaginal sonography. This was confirmed at hysteroscopy where widespread ischemia of the upper uterine surface was noted. This finding was consistent with documentation of low blood flow sonographic Doppler findings.

COMMONLY UNRECOGNIZED UTERINE ANOMALIES

The dominant observation at hysteroscopy was ***extreme pallor and ishemia*** of the uterine fundus. This was seen in the subseptate, anvil, or arcuate uterus. This finding was often missed if one was not aware of the significance of pallor indicating ischemia when viewing the uterine surface.

UTERINE PATHOLOGY

The uterine cavity may have pathology related to postabortal, postpartum, or inflammatory adhesions. Polyps, fibroids, or repeated prior uterine surgeries (including prior C section) may result in significant scarring and/or Asherman's syndrome.

OPERATIVE PROTOCOLS FOR INTRAUTERINE SURGERY

When preparing to correct any of these uterine abnormalities, the surgery was carried out during the proliferative phase of the menstrual cycle. At this time, endometrial repair and healing are at their best.

We used prophylactic antibiotics, together with large doses of estrogen postoperatively as originally described in the 1980s. Over the years, we did not find any form of intrauterine device or catheter, helpful in preventing adhesions during the postoperative phase.

Our impression was that large dose postoperative estrogen therapy was the most important factor preventing postoperative intrauterine scarring. Anecdotally, we assumed that rapid proliferation of endometrium responding to high levels of estradiol would occur before mobilization of the inflammatory reaction that would promulgate adhesions. In recent years, the use of hyaluronic acid gel, placed in the uterus on completion of surgery, has been shown to significantly lower the occurrence of postoperative intrauterine adhesions.

If one was concerned about the extent of the surgery necessary to repair the uterus, then we planned a second look hysteroscopy approximately three to four weeks later in the late proliferative phase of the next cycle. This was not common (5%) but allowed sweeping away early adhesion formation.

POSTOPERATIVE PROTOCOL

The specific postoperative protocol was the administration of estradiol valerate four milligrams every seventy-two hours for five doses, followed by micronized progesterone fifty milligrams twice a day for five days.

The extent of suppression of endometrium with potent synthetic progestins has, I believe, been under estimated.

Personally, I have preferred natural progesterone and have never used progestins postoperatively after repairing a uterus.

As mentioned above, hyaluronic acid gel placed in the uterus, at the end of surgery, has been shown to reduce postoperative adhesions. I would add this gel to the estrogen/progesterone protocol in future surgeries.

ASSESSING POSTSURGICAL UTERINE FUNCTION WITH A SIMULATED TREATMENT CYCLE

When a patient had multiple prior miscarriages and extensive pathology was observed in the uterus, we would follow a complex uterine repair, with a ***simulated "fertile" cycle*** prior to attempting conception.

We administered adequate estrogen and progesterone, over a complete menstrual cycle. We confirmed the dose by checking that the midcycle estradiol level was at least 300 pg/ml before the simulated time of ovulation, and that serum progesterone levels were over 35 ngs/ml systemically in the midluteal phase.

The protocol included oral progesterone 200 milligrams three times a day, vaginal progesterone 100 milligrams two times a day and the systemic progesterone level was invariably equal to or higher than 35 ngs/ml in the peripheral blood.

This ***simulated "fertile" cycle*** was completed with the goal of obtaining a ***day 26 plus "in phase" endometrial biopsy*** scored according to the original description by Georgeanna Seegar Jones using the Noyes, Hertig Rock criteria.

If the biopsy was "in phase" day 26 plus, then we accepted that we had a good functional postoperative outcome.

We then proceeded to accomplish a healthy conception by reproducing all the simulation details. We ensured that the uterus appeared normal on ultrasound at midcycle and that blood levels were consistent with those previously described.

Not uncommonly, prolactin levels rose dramatically when adequate estradiol were accomplished. This event was immediately corrected with bromergocryptine, administered vaginally.

DETAILED ASSESSMENT AND CORRECTION OF FUNDAL ISCHEMIA AT HYSTEROSCOPY

This was accomplished by carefully transecting the fundus approximately a millimeter at a time, and then lowering the intrauterine pressure to see whether or not there was bleeding from the fundal surface.

If the uterine surface was normal, one would see minimal bleeding as soon as one commenced any transection. Further transection was stopped immediately. This was not common in those with a "white" ischemic fundus.

It was more often necessary, to keep transecting, for at least two to three millimeters and sometimes more, before lowering the intrauterine pressure showed some minor fundal bleeding The operation was completed with three to four *ploughing* strokes both anteriorly and posteriorly, using a special 3 mm, two-toothed, ploughing curette.[1]

Finding an ishemic uterine fundus was a most important observation, as many patients had been referred having had a previous hysteroscopy with the anatomy of the uterus documented as normal. The previous surgeon had not been aware of the extreme *"white" ischaemia of the uterine fundus.* Thus, it was not corrected at that time and often resulted in another miscarriage.

---

[1]   Marina Medical Instruments • www.marinamedical.com • Davie, Fl.

HEMATOLOGY

The important causes of abnormal coagulation in pregnancy are known to be anti-phospholipid antibodies, particularly cardiolipin, protein S, Leiden factor, anti-thyroid antibodies, and sticky platelet syndrome.

These abnormalities were all treated with heparin or low molecular weight heparin together with chewable aspirin (salicylate)—81 mg per tab.

Heparin and aspirin were commenced forty-eight hours postovulation. If the patient conceived, anticoagulant therapy was continued right through pregnancy until consideration of delivery. Platelet counts were checked intermittently. The salicylate (81 mg) was discontinued ten days before delivery, and if on low molecular heparin, this was converted to heparin at this time. The heparin was then discontinued approximately twenty-four to thirty-six hours before induction of labor or planned caesarean section.

This anticoagulation protocol was also used in the treatment of patients with elevated natural killer cells (***NK cells***). See below.

Additional testing included antinuclear antibodies ***ANA*** (and its titers), lupus-erythematosis, rheumatoid arthritis, psoriasis, eczema, Sjorgens, asthma, Crohn's disease, irritable bowel syndrome, and endometriosis if noted in the patients history or if there was a family history of these illnesses.

Livedo Reticularis was a common sign in these patients.

A personal or family history of these disorders was always an indication for testing NK cells to exclude that they were not a contributing cause to the patient's recurrent miscarriage problem. The positive rate of NK cells was 25% plus in this group.

NATURAL KILLER CELLS

During the past thirty years, this topic has been an enigma.

It has been extremely controversial to define, interpret, and manage the presence of abnormally high levels of natural killer cells (***NK CELLS***) in pregnant women. Many clinicians have never even checked a NK cell level and absolutely deny any possible relationship to recurrent miscarriage, despite thirty years of peer reviewed literature in the field.

Modern laboratories can test the peripheral blood for NK cells by flow cytometry and they report the percentage of NK cells present.

Normal levels in healthy pregnant women were established +_ 30 years ago at or below 8.5%. A reputable laboratory specializing in these assays can also do in an "in vitro" check of the effects of Interleukin 2 (Il2) stimulation and elevation of the NK cells measured.

If Il2 *stimulates* and elevates a normal level of NK cells to an elevated *abnormal level in a nonpregnant woman*, this rise in the percentage of NK cells killing activity *warns* of the possibility of destructive immunological activity of natural killer cells in pregnancy.

Stated differently, if a patient has a normal percentage of natural killer cells (e.g., 8.5% but IL2 stimulation), takes it to 10%, this is a warning that *the natural killer cells may be activated to cause damage to the pregnancy in this patient.*

In the laboratory that we used[2] a pregnant women's natural killer cells of 8.5% or below were reported as normal. If it was above 9.5%, then the NK cell test was interpreted as abnormally high (positive) IL2 stimulation would document the percentile that natural killer cells may change in pregnancy. If we had a patient with *borderline natural killer cells but elevated Il2 stimulation, we would recheck her natural killer cells as soon as feasible when she was pregnant.* If elevated (now positive), we would treat it accordingly.

These patients were all *placed on heparin and aspirin postovulation.* This was usually continued right until delivery if natural killer cells remained positive. The reason for these anticoagulants is that the NK cells release kinins which cause vascular spasm and thrombosis. This is similar to one of the mechanisms of rejection seen in human transplantation. The low-dose anticoagulation was considered an additional benefit to prevent vascular thrombosis and supplementary to the specific treatment of lowering the percentage of natural killer cells with *Intralipid* (purified soya bean oil and 20% fat emulsion) or *gammaglobulin.*

---

[2] ReproSource • 200 Forest St., 2nd Floor • Marlborough, MA 01752 USA • 800-667-8893 • www.ReproSource.com.

As we have delivered over one thousand patients (over thirty-five years) with a success rate over 80% in patients with positive natural killer cells and an average of five prior losses, I have no doubt that this is a significant clinical disorder.

The most common associations with NK cells were autoimmune disorders including lupus, psoriasis, eczema, asthma, Crohn's disease, ulcerative colitis, IBS, rheumatoid arthritis, and endometriosis in the patient or a family member. ***Livedo Reticularis*** was commonly seen in those with these disorders.

A modern laboratory when documenting positive natural killer cells can also define (in vitro), whether purified soya bean oil with 20% fat emulsion (Intralipid) or gamma globulin would be effective in lowering the natural killer cells in an individual patient (e.g., the report may indicate that the lipid/fat emulsion would lower the NK cells 50% versus gammaglobulin would only lower it 5%, or vice versa).

If there was any doubt of the treatment efficacy in a patient with many losses, and the laboratory had reported that Intralipid would be efficacious, we would use it but remeasure the natural killer cells approximately 10 days later to confirm its therapeutic efficacy. If the NK cells were reduced, we would continue with Soya/fat emulsion (Intralipid) treatment throughout pregnancy. If not, we would cross over to gamma globulin (400 mg per kilogram) given as a slow intravenous infusion over three to four hours. The appropriate treatment was continued till the NK cells were normal in two successive tests. All patients had their ***IGA*** tested before consideration for gammaglobulin therapy.

IMMUNOTHERAPY PROTOCOL FOR ELEVATED NK CELLS

We proceeded to give Intralipid or gammaglobulin approximately ten days prior to conception when the patient was clinically assessed to be in a "good cycle of stimulation" for washed intrauterine insemination (***WIUI***) or in a "well stimulated cycle" for in vitro fertilization. Commenting on the need to be in an "adequate cycle" is important because of the major expenses, (particularly of Gammaglobulin) of these medications. If a cycle was not considered optimal, it was discontinued, and the immunotherapy was saved for a future, more favorable cycle.

Once pregnant, the patient was checked monthly, for the presence or absence of abnormal NK cells.

Three groups of patients emerged.

Those who would return a positive NK cell test every thirty days for ***three months***. Those who remained positive for ***twenty-two to twenty-four weeks***, and the third group would persist with positive natural killer cells every month, ***until delivery.***

In this third group, the gammaglobulin or soya/lipid emulsion (Intralipid) therapy was maintained until the last infusion was given at thirty-four to thirty-five weeks of pregnancy, when it was discontinued, in the knowledge that the soya/lipid emulsion, or gamma globulin, would be effective for a further plus minus four weeks till delivery.

Note: Every patient was screened regarding their level of IGA.

If the ***IGA*** was normal, it was not necessary to check for anti ***IGA*** antibodies. If the ***IGA*** was low, the patient was tested for the presence of IgA antibodies. ***These tests are essential as the presence of low IGA, and positive anti-IGA antibodies is an absolute contraindication to the use of gamma globulin (and indeed all blood products) as such patients have a major risk of anaphylaxis.***

Adhering to these safety criteria, we had no complications other than headache and a few minutes of tachycardia during infusion in some patients.

THE IMPORTANCE OF THE DQ ALPHA PHENOTYPE AND WHEN TO MEASURE IT

In patients with repeated extremely early loss (e.g., immediately post-pregnancy test positive up to eight weeks), we measured the DQ alpha phenotype of both partners. There are two locations on each phenotypic typing (e.g., ***male***—4.1/3.6, ***female***—3.8/2.6). This would be an acceptable result. However, if you have matches between male and female phenotypes, this is reported to cause more aggressive immuno-rejection reactions. This fortunately uncommon event is an indication for the use of gamma-globulin. A complete match of both partners (e.g., 4.1/4.1–4.1/4.1) is not compatible with a viable outcome. This has been reported as an indication for donor sperm or donor oocytes from one with a dissimilar phenotype.

RECONSIDERATION OF THE MEASUREMENT OF NK CELLS

As many reviews of *still birth* record a *40% incidence of "unexplained" causes*, yet the Obstetric community continue to shun measurement of NK cells up to this time.

Should we be looking for immunological natural killer cell syndromes?

They may cause microvascular clotting, Abruptio-placenta, *IUGR*, and sudden stillbirth in a significant number of patients.

Prospective double-blind studies should be established regarding the presence or absence of *NK cells* in these assessed as high-risk obstetric patients.

HCG
Human Chorionic Gonadotropin

This medication should possibly also be looked at again in double-blind prospective, strictly controlled trials. It was used extensively in the late 1960s for recurrent miscarriage on the basis of its luteotropic, trophoblastotropic, and immunosuppressive qualities.

COMMENT

When reviewing the multiple patients presenting with recurrent miscarriage, we found many factors which collectively were the cause of the problem. *One of the major issues was the ovulatory quantity of hormones particularly in older patients*, who, in addition to their age factor, had come through major stresses of life, had a low *BMI*, excessive athleticism, nutritional disorders, or prolonged estrogen progesterone suppression.

Many of these women (when their records were available) tended to have lower hormonal levels prior to ovulation and poor luteal phase cycles were noted in their prior conception(s).

Thus, a thirty-eight-year-old presenting with recurrent miscarriage, although already handicapped by a significant percentage of aneuploidy (+_40%), would commence pregnancy with low levels of estrogen and progesterone and inadequately prepared endometrium. This often unrecognized issue would be added to any other causes diagnosed.

The history would reveal E2 levels of _+_150 pgs at ovulation and +_ 80 pgs during the luteal phase. This was commonly associated with progesterone levels of 6 to 10 ngs /ml during the luteal phase of their cycles.

We considered this a significant factor and ensured that every patient commenced pregnancy with adequate estrogen in the proliferative phase, and adequate progesterone and estrogen, during the luteal phase of the cycle of conception.

This concept is not new for, ever since the advent of the birth control pill, patients were usually encouraged to wait two or three cycles after discontinuing their hormonal contraception before attempting to conceive. This was due to the possibility of inadequate ovulatory cycles that may occur in the first cycles posthormonal suppression. It was thought that the hypothalamic pituitary axis would require some time to regain its normal function. With this in mind, we ensured adequate hormonal levels in the cycle of conception. *One cannot stress enough, that individualized care was a prerequisite to effect these protocols.*

PLANNING FOR "MONO-FOLLICULAR OVULATION"

The clinical technique used to achieve single follicular ovulation (in almost every cycle) was to wait till there was a *dominant* follicle, +_ day 6–7, from the first day of menses, in those with twenty-eight day cycles.

Follicular dominance was closer to day 10 to 13 in those with *PCOS* and associated longer cycles. Once a dominant follicle was confirmed, we would stimulate and augment the cycle with human menopausal gonadotropin *(FSH/LH)* as required. We also augmented with oral E2 and oral and vaginal progesterone if needed in the luteal phase of the cycle of conception.

HCG-(5000 IUs) was given at midcycle in every cycle if at all possible. This would ensure ovulation and the *physical release of the oocyte* in over 95% of cycles.

HCG was also given to enhance the luteal phase production of hormones, and because it is also trophoblastotropic and a positive hormone known to promote implantation. This augmentation of ovulation in the cycle of conception (once a dominant follicle was confirmed) resulted in mono follicular ovulation in over 95% of cases. The additional 5% may have had +_ two follicles, and 5% of this group conceived twins.

CERVICAL INCOMPETENCE

In the past three decades, the management of cervical incompetence has also become increasingly controversial.

With a history of sudden, unexplained painless losses (occasionally earlier), but usually after eighteen to twenty weeks of gestation, a clear-cut diagnosis of cervical incompetence may be established. This is confirmed by admission of a Hegar 8 dilator in the nonpregnant patient's cervix, combined with seeing marked funneling of the lower uterus and cervix at hysterosalpingogram. These definitive findings confirm a diagnosis of cervical incompetence. ***This may be uncommon but when seen, confirms the diagnosis.***

As the uterus grows actively till approximately eighteen to twenty weeks of gestation, there is no particular pressure on the cervix at this time. Thereafter, the uterus stretches with increasing intrauterine pressure from twenty weeks; thus, not having prospectively diagnosed cervical incompetence in this kind of patient is often regretted. For watching the growing uterus before twenty weeks may encourage a false sense of security about the cervix, the intrauterine pressure rises, the cervix suddenly dilates, and the pregnancy is lost.

When the history of such a patient is this clear-cut, it is my opinion that once euploidy (normal genetics and chromosomes) is confirmed at eight to nine weeks, then a cerclage should be placed in early pregnancy.

In days gone by, we knew that many chromosomal abnormalities would result in early loss so that we waited till twelve completed weeks before inserting a cerclage. This became a tradition which I do not think is necessary at this time.

Early placement of a cervical cerclage is technically far easier to insert at approximately ten to twelve weeks of pregnancy. We used polypropylene placed as a double or triple cerclage. My impression anecdotally was that there were far less infective complications using this method. Recent data at other gynecologic surgical sites confirms these thoughts.

We were also highly proactive and conservative with respect to the patients' perioperative and postoperative management.

Perioperatively, the patient was given intramuscular progesterone 100 mg on the morning of Cerclage, 100 mg in the evening, and 50 mg twice a day for the next forty-eight hours. She was also ***kept in bed for three to four days*** after the procedure and her physical activities reduced significantly. When mersilene or an alternative tape is used, it is essential that it should be buried. As being hydrophilic, it appears to be associated with a higher risk of infection.

In recent years, the advent of transabdominal laprascopic cerclage, particularly in those who have had a failed a vaginal procedure, has clearly been a major advance in this field.

SUMMARY

Recurrent miscarriage remains a major problem causing great emotional and physical morbidity in a significant number of patients.

This section provides an anecdotal perspective of a clinician's experience over fifty years in the diagnosis and management of this problem.

As mentioned, the patients had already consulted two to three physicians and were referred after repeated failures, with an average of five prior losses.

This was extremely important as it influenced the type of patient seen. They may represent a ***highly skewed and selective group seen much later in their care.***

It was important to ***make no assumptions re the most obvious cause, but to complete all the testing reviewed.***

There were commonly at least three to four factors in each couple.

Very few couples had the exact same diagnosis or treatment protocol.

It was thus critical that they each be assessed as unique and individual.

It was also essential to document blood levels in the individual. Different patients required significantly different amounts of medication to attain adequate blood levels. This applies to their estrogen and progesterone requirements in their simulated and actual treatment cycles

When we establish evidence-based, uniform protocols gathered by meta-analysis of mass statistical observation, *individual patient care may be compromised.* He or she may not fit the universal protocol rigid format.

Is also essential that the physician and nurses caring for these patients are sensitively cognizant of the emotional and psychiatric welfare of these subjects.

They have been through extreme trauma, and have their own post multiple miscarriages, traumatic syndromes. Clearly, they need emotional backup at all times during the diagnosis and subsequent management of their problems. Seeking detailed *individualized diagnosis and management does I believe result in the maximum yield of healthy viable babies* in this type of cohort of patients.

The opinions expressed in this booklet are purely those of the author. They do not formally direct specific treatment options or methods. These thoughts should be reviewed by all couples with their physicians, who will direct their own treatment strategies. This booklet explains basic methods and should be a guide to provide reassuring direction in your care. These diagnosis and treatment techniques were formulated by synthesis of evidence based writing in the literature over the past fifty years. They were applied to my own patients, under my care.

Glossary

ADHESIONS

Bands of scar tissue that may be present in or over any organ or tissue in the abdomen. Such adhesions may be present in the uterus, over or in the fallopian tubes and over or in the ovaries. It is usually necessary to surgically remove these adhesions to free the underlying healthy tissue or organs trapped by these fibrous scars so that they can function normally.

ADRENOCORTICOTROPIC HORMONE (ACTH)

The hormonal that stimulates the adrenal cortex to produce cortisol and other hormones from the adrenal glands.

ANTI-IGA ANTIBODIES

There are an absolute contraindication to the administration of intravenous GAMMA GLOBULIN as the risks of anaphylaxis are extremely high.

ANTI-MULLERIAN HORMONE (AMH)

The hormone that is secreted by cells around the small follicles of the ovary. The lower the number, the lower the AMH. Thus, a lower number of residual follicles will be seen with a low AMH. This is one of the hormones used as an indication of the patient's ovarian reserve. There should be more than eight follicles on day 3 of the cycle, and less than four follicles is associated with a low ovarian reserve.

ASSISTED REPRODUCTIVE TECHNOLOGY (ART)

Preparation of sperm includes in vitro fertilization, intra cytoplasmic sperm injection (ICSI) embryo culture, embryo transfer, freezing (cryo preservation) of sperm, eggs, and embryo preimplantation genetic diagnosis.

DILATATION AND CURETTAGE (D&C)

In this minor surgery, the cervix is dilated so that a suction or gentle scrapping instrument (curette) can be passed through the cervix to the inside of the uterus, which is then gently scraped and cleansed with this instrument.

ENDOMETRIOSIS

A condition characterized by tissue resembling the endometrial lining of the uterus (endometrium) found outside the normal lining of the uterus. Endometriosis is commonly found behind the uterus, deposited on the utero-sacral ligaments and around or on the bladder, bowel, and the fallopian tubes. It is also found within or on the surface of the ovaries. Endometriosis lesions may cause recurrent severe pelvic pain and is commonly related to infertility.

ESTRADIOL

This is the primary female sex hormone secreted by the ovary, responsible for growth of the female organs and reproduction. The vagina, endometrium, uterus, and the maintenance of the cervical and tubal secretions. It also plays a role in tubal muscular function. It is the major hormone involved in the regulation of the female reproductive cycle. Most is made by the ovaries, but the adrenal glands and fat cells may also secrete small amounts. It plays a role in preserving the oocyte (eggs) of a woman. It is important in breast development and maintenance of secondary sexual characters of the female.

FOLLICLE-STIMULATING HORMONE (FSH)
AND LUTEINIZING HORMONE (LH)

FSH stimulates the ovaries and testicles. In the female, it stimulates follicular growth in the ovaries and subsequent production of estrogens and progesterone with the assistance of LH from the corpus luteum. In the male, FSH is dominantly involved in the production of spermatozoa. LH is dominant in stimulating the interstitial cells (within the testicles) to produce testosterone.

GALACTORRHEA

Abnormal production of milk from the breast. Prolactin elevation in a nonpregnant woman causes abnormal hormonal function and interferes with ovulation and may cause infertility and miscarriage.

HUMAN MENOPAUSAL GONADOTROPIN (HMG)

This is an injectable hormone contained in seventy-five international units of FSH combined with seventy-five international units of LH in a single ampule. The preparation is manufactured, from menopausal urine which is purified, concentrated, and specifically cleansed by fractionation to ensure a safe product for subcutaneous or intramuscular injection. It is also available prepared by recombinant technology. This injection in various doses resembles, replaces, or augments the natural levels of FSH and LH released from the pituitary gland to stimulate the ovaries.

INSULIN RESISTANCE

This is a condition not uncommonly seen in women with polycystic ovarian syndrome. Insulin appears to be less functionally efficient. Higher levels of insulin are required to control the level of sugar in the blood. Insulin resistance may occur prior to diabetes but is not diabetes itself. This problem, often related to polycystic ovaries, is associated with an unhealthy environment for the oocytes (eggs). One attempts to lower the insulin by reducing carbohydrate intake with an appropriate low carbohydrate diet and exercise. If these measures of diet and exercise do not lower insulin, the patient may require medication (commonly glucophage—metformin) to assist in this metabolic problem.

INTRA-CYTOPLASMIC SPERM INJECTION (ICSI)

A single sperm is placed in an egg. This is completed at in vitro fertilization under the operating microscope.

PITUITARY GLAND

This gland is situated beneath the brain and centrally behind the eyes. It controls all the basic hormones of the body. Growth, thyroid, parathyroid, adrenals, ovaries, testicles.

PRE-IMPLANTATION GENETIC DIAGNOSIS (PGD)

Ruling out chromosomal and genetic abnormalities of an embryo. Basic technique is to take a cell from the embryo and send it for chromosomal and genetic analysis. The resulting normal embryo(s) examined are usually kept and maintained frozen at -196 degrees Celsius (in liquid nitrogen) for transfer to the patient's uterus in subsequently prepared adequate hormonally monitored transfer cycles.

PROGESTERONE

This is a hormone secreted primarily from the corpus luteum of the ovary. It plays a major role in preparing the endometrium (inner lining of the uterus) for pregnancy. It is the dominant hormone ensuring relaxation of the uterine muscles in later pregnancy. During pregnancy after the first trimester, most is produced by the placenta. It is also produced by the adrenal glands usually in lesser quantities.

PROLACTIN

A hormone from the pituitary which stimulates the breasts in preparation for breast milk in pregnancy. When elevated in a nonpregnant woman, this may suppress ovulation, cause abnormal hormone function, infertility or miscarriage. Usually easy controlled with pills that are dopamine agonists.

THYROID-STIMULATING HORMONE (TSH)

This hormone controls the activity of the thyroid gland. It is usually high when the thyroid function is low. It is usually low when the thyroid function is high.

WASHED INTRAUTERINE HYDRO INSEMINATION "HYDRO INSEMINATION"

This technique was originally proposed in the early 1980s. Routine preparation of the sperm is completed using an optimal semen friendly culture medium. After three washes, the sperm is placed in *3 to 4 ml of warm culture medium* in a nontoxic 5 ml disposable syringe. The syringe is placed at the cervix via a "Christmas tree" fitting to a non-toxic rubber cone. The cone is placed gently but firmly against the cervical o.s. (after cleansing away the mucus in the routine manner), and the sperm is *hydrotubated slowly via the uterus into the fallopian tubes.* This method was associated with higher pregnancy rates in the 1980s, and we have continued to use it.

QUESTIONAIRE FEMALE

Name (Female): ____

Age at onset of menstruation: _____________

Menstrual cycle: ☐ Regular ☐ Irregular

    Days bleeding/days between cycles: _______________

    (For example: 5 days bleeding/28 days between → 5/28)

    Pain with periods: ☐ Yes ☐ No

    Treatment for this pain: _______________________________

    Bleeding between periods: ☐ Yes ☐ No

    Bleeding after intercourse ☐ Yes ☐ No

Mother's age at menopause: _______________________

Numbers of years you have been attempting conception: _____________

Number of pregnancies: _____________

    Live births: _______________

    Still births: _______________

    Miscarriages: _______________

    Tubal pregnancies: _____________

    Date: Right tube: _____________

    Left tube: _____________

    Terminations: _______________________

Prior history of birth control method:

    Type: ____

    Duration: ____

History of pelvic infection: ☐ Yes ☐ No

Previous sterilization: ☐ Yes ☐ No

Request for sterilization reversal: ☐ Yes ☐ No

Reason for seeking reversal: _______________________________________

____

Any vaginal discharges: ☐ Yes ☐ No

    Treatment: _______________________________________

Urinary Difficulties: ☐ Burning ☐ Increased frequency

    ☐ Prior urinary infections, treatment: _______________________

Regular bowel habits: ☐ Yes ☐ No

    ☐ Constipation ☐ Diarrhea

    Treatment: _______________________________________

Pain accompanying bowel movements: ☐ Yes ☐ No

    Related to menses: ☐ Yes ☐ No

Frequency of sexual intercourse: _____________ # times per week

    Painful intercourse: ☐ Yes ☐ No

    Superficial pain Deep (inside lower abdomen)

    Use of vaginal lubricants: ☐ Yes ☐ No

    Use of douche: ☐ Yes ☐ No; frequency: _____________

    Patient Information/Questionnaire

Name (Female): ____

Weight: __________ Has there been any major weight loss or gain: ☐ Yes ☐ No

Reason why: ____

Height: ______ Exercise: ______# hours per week

Skin problems/acne: ☐ Yes ☐ No Treatment: _______________________________

Excessive hair: ☐ Facial ☐ Abdominal ☐ Inner thighs

Any milky discharge from breasts: ☐ Yes ☐ No

Any problems with headaches: ☐ Yes ☐ No

Are you frequently hot or cold (circle one) when people around you are comfortable.

Visual problems: ☐ Eyeglasses ☐ Contacts

Difficulties in peripheral vision: ☐ Yes ☐ No

Any heart palpitations: ☐ Yes ☐ No

Any Known Drug Allergies: ____

Any Known Drug Reactions: ____

Smoking: ☐ Yes ☐ No Number per day: ____________

Alcohol: ☐ Yes ☐ No Number per week: ____________

per month: ____________

per day: ____________

Recreational Drugs: ☐ Yes ☐ No Name of Drug or Substance____________________

<u>**Personal Medical History**</u>:   Comment

Diabetes	☐ Yes	☐ No	______________________
High blood pressure	☐ Yes	☐ No	______________________
Heart disease	☐ Yes	☐ No	______________________
Thyroid problems	☐ Yes	☐ No	______________________
Breast cancer	☐ Yes	☐ No	______________________
Other cancers	☐ Yes	☐ No	______________________
Autoimmune disorders	☐ Yes	☐ No	______________________
Kidney disease	☐ Yes	☐ No	______________________
Blood clotting disorders	☐ Yes	☐ No	______________________
Asthma	☐ Yes	☐ No	______________________
Hepatitis or other liver disease	☐ Yes	☐ No	______________________
Anemia	☐ Yes	☐ No	______________________
Eating disorder	☐ Yes	☐ No	______________________
Sexually transmitted disease	☐ Yes	☐ No	______________________
Psychiatric disorders	☐ Yes	☐ No	______________________
Genetic disorders	☐ Yes	☐ No	______________________

Proprietary information of National Fertility Center / Cohen Center Dallas, Texas
(CANNOT BE REPRODUCED WITHOUT THE WRITTEN CONSENT OF THIS ENTITY)

Name (Female): ____

Personal Medical History (continued):

Birth defects	☐ Yes	☐ No	_______________________
Other health problems	☐ Yes	☐ No	_______________________

Medication(s) you currently take and dosage(s) per day:_______________________________________

____

List any herbs you currently take and dosage(s) per day:_______________________________________

____

Family history: Comment

Diabetes	☐ Yes	☐ No	_______________________
High Blood Pressure	☐ Yes	☐ No	_______________________
Heart Disease	☐ Yes	☐ No	_______________________
Thyroid Problems	☐ Yes	☐ No	_______________________
Breast Cancer	☐ Yes	☐ No	_______________________
Other reproductive or genital cancers	☐ Yes	☐ No	_______________________
Autoimmune Disease	☐ Yes	☐ No	_______________________
Downs Syndrome	☐ Yes	☐ No	_______________________
Mental Retardation	☐ Yes	☐ No	_______________________
Birth Defects	☐ Yes	☐ No	_______________________

Genetic Screening Tests:

Are either you or your husband from:

1) Eastern European Jewish ancestry?   ☐ Yes   ☐ No

   If yes, have you been tested for Tay Sachs carrier status? _____________

2) African American ancestry?   ☐ Yes   ☐ No

   If yes, have you been tested for sickle cell trait? _____________

3) Italian, Greek, or Mediterranean ancestry?   ☐ Yes   ☐ No

   If yes, have you been tested for beta thalassemia minor? _____________

4) Philippine or Southeast Asian ancestry?   ☐ Yes   ☐ No

   If yes, have you been tested for alpha thalassemia minor? _____________

Name (Female): ____

<u>**Previous testing and treatments**</u>:

<u>**Name of Test**</u>	<u>**Date**</u>	<u>**Results**</u>
Rubella (German measles)	__________	____________________________
Post Coital test	__________	____________________________
Endometrial biopsy	__________	____________________________
Prolactin	__________	____________________________
DHEAS	__________	____________________________
TSH	__________	____________________________
Progesterone	__________	____________________________
Testosterone	__________	____________________________
Blood type & Rh	__________	____________________________
Last pap smear	__________	____________________________
Chlamydia culture	__________	____________________________
Sperm antibody test	__________	____________________________
Day 3: FSH	__________	____________________________
LH	__________	____________________________
E2	__________	____________________________
Other	__________	____________________________

Have you ever had: Hysterosalpingogram (x-ray) ☐ Yes ☐ No

Date: _______ Results: ____________________________

Have you ever had: Laparoscopy ☐ Yes ☐ No

Date: _______ Results: ____________________________

Date: _______ Results: ____________________________

Hysteroscopy ☐ Yes ☐ No

Date: _______ Results: ____________________________

Have you ever had: Artificial Insemination (Husband's sperm): ☐ Yes ☐ No

Artificial Insemination (Donor sperm): ☐ Yes ☐ No

Washed Intrauterine Insemination: ☐ Yes ☐ No

Gamete Intra-fallopian Transfer: ☐ Yes ☐ No Date: _______

In Vitro Fertilization: ☐ Yes ☐ No Date: _______

Name (Female): ____

Have you ever used:

Clomiphene Citrate (Clomid or Serophene):	☐ Yes	☐ No
For how long: ________________________		
HCG injections:	☐ Yes	☐ No
For how long: ________________________		
Fertility (ovarian stimulation) injections:	☐ Yes	☐ No Type:__________
For how long: ________________________		
Progesterone supplementation:	☐ Yes	☐ No
For how long: ________________________		
GnRH agonists (Lupron):	☐ Yes	☐ No
For how long: ________________________		
Danocrine or Danazol:	☐ Yes	☐ No
For how long: ________________________		
Bromocryptine (Parlodel):	☐ Yes	☐ No
For how long: ________________________		

Please list previous surgeries or hospital admissions (date and procedure), including previous laparotomies:

____

____

____

____

____

____

Please give a personal summary (treatment goals and objectives):_____________________

____

____

____

____

____

____

                                   Patient Information/Questionnaire

Proprietary information of National Fertility Center / Cohen Center Dallas, Texas
(CANNOT BE REPRODUCED WITHOUT THE WRITTEN CONSENT OF THIS ENTITY)

QUESTIONAIRE MALE

Name (Male): ____

Number of children fathered: _____________

Number of ejaculations/week: _____________

Blood type/Rh: _____________

Number of years attempting conception with this partner: _____________

Any urinary difficulties or infections: ☐ Yes   ☐ No

Treatment: ____

Any prior testicular injuries: ☐ Yes   ☐ No

Any prior inguinal or testicular surgeries, e.g. hernia repair, varicocele: ☐ Yes   ☐ No

    Year of operation: _____________

Regular bowel habits: ☐ Yes   ☐ No

    ☐ Constipation   ☐ Diarrhea

    Treatment: ____

Frequency of sexual intercourse: _______# times per week

    Decreased sexual desire: ☐ Yes   ☐ No

    Painful ejaculations: ☐ Yes   ☐ No

Weight: _______   Has there been any major weight loss or gain: ☐ Yes   ☐ No

    Reason why: ____

Skin problems/Acne: ☐ Yes   ☐ No

    Treatment: ____

Any problems with headaches: ☐ Yes   ☐ No
    Treatment:

Any visual problems: ☐ Eyeglasses   ☐ Contacts

    Difficulties in peripheral vision: ☐ Yes   ☐ No

Any problems with anxiety attacks: ☐ Yes   ☐ No

Any heart palpitations: ☐ Yes   ☐ No

Any known drug allergies: ____

Any know drug reactions: ____

Name (Male):____

Smoking: ☐ Yes ☐ No Number per day: _____________
Alcohol: ☐ Yes ☐ No Number per week: ___________
                       per month: ___________
                       per day: ___________
Recreational Drugs: ☐ Yes ☐ No Name of Drug or Substance______________________

Vocational Hazards: ☐ Gases ☐ Toxins ☐ Chemicals ☐ Insecticides ☐ Other poisons
What type?____

Personal Medical History:

			Comment
Diabetes	☐ Yes	☐ No	_______
Kidney disease	☐ Yes	☐ No	_______
Asthma	☐ Yes	☐ No	_______
High blood pressure	☐ Yes	☐ No	_______
Hepatitis or other liver disease	☐ Yes	☐ No	_______
Sexually transmitted disease	☐ Yes	☐ No	_______
Psychiatric disorders	☐ Yes	☐ No	_______
Genetic disorders	☐ Yes	☐ No	_______
Birth defects	☐ Yes	☐ No	_______
Other health problems	☐ Yes	☐ No	_______

Medication(s) you currently take and dosage(s) per day:________________________________
____

List any herbs you currently take and dosage(s) per day:_________________________________
____

Family history:

			Comment
Diabetes	☐ Yes	☐ No	_______
Testicular Cancer	☐ Yes	☐ No	_______
Prostate Cancer	☐ Yes	☐ No	_______
Downs Syndrome	☐ Yes	☐ No	_______
Mental Retardation	☐ Yes	☐ No	_______
Birth Defects	☐ Yes	☐ No	_______

Revised 11/02   Patient Information/Questionnaire

Name (Male): ____

Do you wear: ☐ briefs/jockey underwear   ☐ boxer shorts

Do you use hot tubs or jacuzzis: ☐ Yes   ☐ No

Have you ever had:

Semen analysis: ☐ Yes   ☐ No
Date: _______   Result: ____

Hamster test: ☐ Yes   ☐ No
Date: _______   Result: ____

Sperm antibody test: ☐ Yes   ☐ No
Date: _______   Result: ____

Have you ever been on any medication to increase your sperm count or motility: ☐ Yes   ☐ No
Type of medication: ____

Please list previous surgeries or hospital admissions (date and procedure):

____
____
____
____
____
____

Please give a personal summary (treatment goals and objectives):_______________

____
____
____
____
____
____
____

Proprietary information of National Fertility Center / Cohen Center Dallas, Texas
(CANNOT BE REPRODUCED WITHOUT THE WRITTEN CONSENT OF THIS ENTITY)

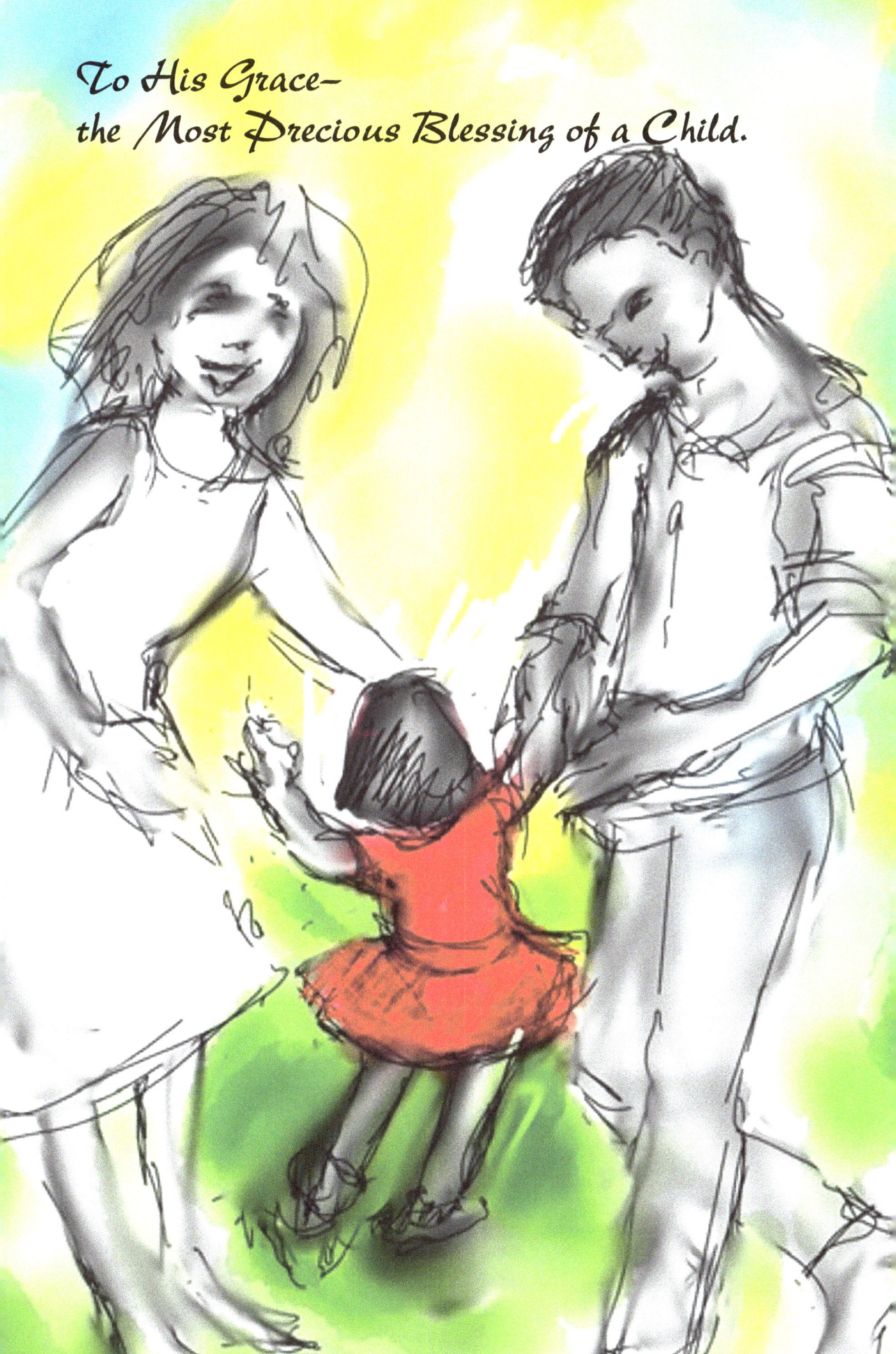
To His Grace–
the Most Precious Blessing of a Child.

About the Author

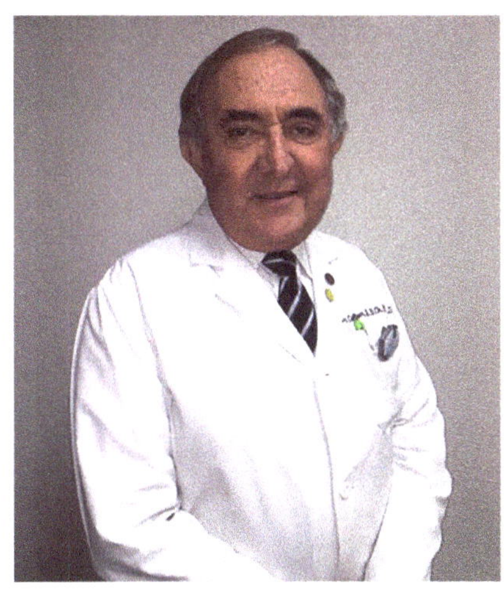

Dr. Brian M. Cohen, MB., Ch.B., M.D. (post-doctoral), F.A.C.O.G., F.R.C.O.G. (Lond.), F.C.O.G. (S.A.) F.I.C.S., F.A.C.E., Board Certified etc. by the American Board of Obstetrics and Gynecology and the Sub Speciality of Reproductive Endocrinology and Infertility.

Dr. Brian Cohen has practiced gynecology for over fifty years.

Early in his career, he was a pioneer in tubal surgery, microsurgery, and vascular tubal transplantation.

His transplantation research over four years earned him the Brontë Stewart Award for the most meritorious postdoctoral thesis at the University of Cape Town in 1975.

Dr. Cohen then completed a fellowship in reproductive endocrinology under Drs. Peter Baillie and Maurice Katz at the University of Cape Town. Drs. Katz and Cohen were among the first to document the hormonal changes of Wedge Resection in Polycystic Ovaries.

He also studied with Professor Philip Rhodes and Mr. Ronald Taylor at the University of London St. Thomas Hospital.

He was associate professor–head of Reproductive Surgery at the University Tennessee in Memphis, working with Dr. James R Givens, associate professor at the University of Michigan with Professor Alan Beer and completed a second fellowship of reproductive endocrinology at Case Western University with Dr. Brian Little in Cleveland, Ohio.

He has been Clinical Professor in the Department of Obstetrics and Gynecology at The University of Texas Southwestern Medical Center since his appointment in 1987.

He is a past president of the AAGL-MIGS—the largest laparoscopic and minimal invasive gynecological surgical society in the world. Always on the cutting edge of new developments in fertility treatment, he taught over three thousand US gynecologists, tubal-microsurgery, operative laparoscopy, hysteroscopy, and vaginal sonography.

He has over fifty years of experience with the use of ovulation induction agents. At one stage, he directed the semenology laboratories at the University of Cape Town and later at the University of Tennessee. Although lecturing on many of these topics throughout the world, he has always been at the bedside, personally taking care of his patients. He has brought all this cumulative study, practice, and experience together to synthesize this simple booklet.